Homoeopathic Treatment of Diarrhoea, Dysentery, Cholera Morbus, and the Cholera: With Repertories for These Diseases

Benjamin Franklin Joslin

HOMŒOPATHIC TREATMENT

OF

DIARRHŒA, DYSENTERY, CHOLERA MORBUS,

AND THE

CHOLERA.

WITH

REPERTORIES FOR THESE DISEASES.

BY B. F. JOSLIN, M. D.

Second Edition.

New-York:
WM. RADDE, 322 BROADWAY.

1849.

H. Ludwig & Co., Printers,
70 Vesey St., N. Y.

CONTENTS.

CHAP. VIII.—SYMPTOMS AND TREATMENT OF THE STAGES OF THE CHOLERA.

CHAP. IX.—CHOLERA REPERTORY, *for* SYMPTOMS AND GROUPS, *with the values of the medicines distinguished.*

CHAP. X.—GASTRIC AND INTESTINAL REPERTORY; *Auxiliary to the Cholera Repertory, and adapted to Vomiting, Diarrhœa, Cholera Infantum and Dysentery.*

INTRODUCTION.

The Cholera will re-appear soon, and spread extensively, and a book on its causes and prevention, and especially its treatment, be required by the profession. The author has aimed to prepare, for the use of Homœopathic physicians, a portable treatise, so systematic and so full, as to enable them to find, with facility, the remedy for every curable case of this disease.

It will offer the advantage of a threefold arrangement of the principal medicines; viz., with reference, 1st, to the varieties; 2d, to the stages; and 3d, to the symptoms as arranged in the Cholera Repertory. The repertories will give the book a permanent value, as a pocket companion, in treating the more frequent complaints of summer.

It is believed, that physicians will find in the plain rules for prevention, preliminary, treatment and nursing, a safe and convenient basis for instructions to be given to the families in which they practise.

As it is believed that many of our brethren who are at present Allœopathic, will be induced to treat the Cholera Homœopathically, the more important rules of treatment are given in a more particular and elementary form than would be necessary for an experienced Homœopathic practitioner. If any one should fail in some of his first attempts at Homœopathic treatment, in any curable malady, the fault would not be in the law, but in its administration. Let him not impute to Homœopathy the results of his own ignorance, indolence or haste. No man of merely moderate intellect, industry and attainments, should enter the profession, nor should any physician consider the faithful study of a case too onerous, when human life depends on the correctness of his prescription. The following are the requirement and injunction of Hahnemann: "To the physician, whose province it is to vanquish the disease that brings its victim to the very borders of corporeal dissolution, and to produce, as it were, a second creation of life—a greater work than almost all the other much-vaunted performances of mankind—to him Nature, in all her wide expanse, with all her sources and productions, must lie open. * * * Let all hold aloof from this most pious, this noblest of all secular professions, who are deficient in mind, in patient thought, in the requisite knowledge, or in tender philanthropy and a sense of duty."

The author has taken some portions of the 1st and 2d chapters, from his own paper on "Epidemic Cholera," published in the "Transactions of the Medical Society of the State of New-York." As an Allœopathic physician, he was familiar with the Cholera of 1832 and '4. Those prescriptions which succeeded best with him, were those which were most nearly Homœopathic. He remembers patients restored from collapse and cured, by camphor. He has recently tested the proper Homœopathic treatment, in some severe cases of Asiatic Cholera, and in others of a mixed character; besides securing by prophylactics some persons exposed. But in giving a plan of treatment, he has not relied on his own limited experience and unaided reflections, but endeavored to describe that which, both as to remedies and attenuations, has been found most successful by the great body of Homœopathic physicians; and for this purpose has consulted all the good treatises on this pestilence which were accessible.

A pamphlet published at Paris, in the French language, by F. F. Quin, M. D., President of the British Homœopathic Society, is probably the best practical work that has hitherto been written on the Cholera. The author of this book believed that he could not do a better service to the English reader, than by translating every important part of that, except in cases in which he had introduced similar ideas in other language or in a different connexion. Most of the symptoms of the seventh chapter are thus taken, and constitute nearly all that has been merely translated.

Much labor and reflection have been given to Chapter IX. In composing this Cholera Repertory, the claims of each medicine which has reputation in this disease, has been examined, for almost every symptom, in the Symptomen Codex of Jahr, or the Materia Medica of Hahnemann, or in both.* The Homœopathic Materia Medica is the true test of the correctness of conclusions drawn from Clinical experience; indeed, it was originally the only guide to that practice which was attended with such splendid results in 1832. It was Hahnemann's confidence in this, and in his law of cure, that enabled him to publish the plan on which this fearful malady was successfully combated.

With his usual sagacity, he pointed out the true prophylactics, and all the most important curatives, when this pestilence had not fallen under his own observation. Having discovered and demonstrated a universal, unerring, and everlasting law in medicine, he was prepared to encounter the strangest forms of disease as though they were familiar.

The law is *similia similibus curantur*, like are cured by like; or (to expand this brief and elliptical aphorism) diseases are cured by medicines which tend to excite affections similar to the diseases themselves. From the Greek, ὅμοιον πάθος, (homoion pathos, affectus similis,) the Latin term Homœopathia, and the English Homœopathy, are derived.

* Chapter X., is compiled chiefly from Jahr, with certain modifications, but almost always with the preservation of the emphasis of the French edition.

We frequently hear persons who have no experience in Homœopathy—or who at most have seen its effect in Chronic cases,—saying, I would not dare to trust it if I were very sick, with a dangerous and rapid disease. I should want something that would act powerfully and quickly. A potentized medicine selected in accordance with the Homœopathic law, is that very thing. Thousands of physicians know it to be such; and that in their own former Allœopathic practice, and in that of their brethren of the old school, no violent and rapid diseases have been cured as surely and promptly as they now cure them by the Homœopathic method.

Homœopathy has been eminently successful in dangerous *Epidemic* diseases, caused by some subtle poison in the atmosphere, whether communicated from the sick, or from any other source. In the Typhus Fever, that prevailed lately to some extent in this city, the Homœopathic physicians demonstrated the truth and power of their system, by the success of appropriate remedies, and especially of Rhus Radicans. A destructive form of this epidemic Typhus, broke out in the routed army of Napoleon, during his disastrous retreat from Russia, and spread from it through several countries, baffling the skill of all, except the Homœopathic Physicians. In the effects of infinitessimal doses they saw the verification of the maxim, "die milde Macht ist gross," the mild power is great.

Large doses are not required to cure any disease whatever. Attenuation, whilst it weakens and ultimately nullifies poisons, as such, is in almost every substance essential to the full development of medicinal power; and, in some substances, no medicinal power whatever is manifested until the substance is rendered extremely dilute.

This book will contain abundant experimental evidence of the efficacy of attenuated medicines in the treatment of Cholera. The great success of European physicians in the treatment of the Asiatic Cholera of 1832, was due to the use of attenuated medicines, as well as to the law of similitude, which regulated their administration.

The following is a *list of the Cholera Medicines*, with the proper attenuations.

Names.			*Abbreviations.*
Aconitum, 24th attenuation;		"	Acon.^{24} *
Arsenicum, 30th;	"	"	*Ars.*^{30}
Belladonna, 30th;	"	"	Bell.^{30}
Bryonia, 30th;	"	"	Bry.^{30}
Camphora, Tinct. & 3d,	"	"	Camph.^{0} & ^{3}
Cantharis, 30th;	"	"	Canth.^{30}
Carbo Vegetabilis, 30th;	"	"	*Carb. v.*^{30}
Chamomilla, 30th;	"	"	Cham.^{30}
Cicuta, 30th;	"	"	Cic.^{30}
Cinchona, 12th;	"	"	Chin.^{12}
CUPRUM, 30th;	"	"	CUPR.^{30}
Acidum hydrocyanicum, 30th;		"	Hydrocy.^{30}
Ipecacuanha, 3d,	"	"	*Ipec.*^{3}
Jatropha, 12th;	"	"	*Jat.*^{12}
Laurocerasus, 12th;	"	"	Laur^{12}
Mercurius vivus, 12th:	"	"	Merc.^{12}
Natrum muriaticum, 12th;	"	"	Natr. m.^{12}
Nux vomica, 30th;	"	"	Nux,^{30}
PHOSPHORUS, 30th;	"	"	PHOS.^{30}
PHOSPHORI ACIDUM, 3d, & 30th;		"	PHOS. AC.^{3} & ^{30}
Rhus radicans, 30th;	"	"	R. rad.^{30}
Secale cornutum, 12th;	"	"	*Sec.*^{12}
Stramonium, 12th;	"	"	Stram.^{12}
Sulphur, 30th;	"	"	Sulph.^{30}
Tartarus emeticus, 12th;	"	"	Tart.^{12}
VERATRUM, 12th & 30th;		"	VERAT.^{12} & ^{30}

The distinctions of type, refer to the more or less frequent demand for these medicines, in the disease proper, but not

* This elevated location of the figures in the last column, promotes brevity and prevents ambiguity, where other figures or words follow. It is also appropriate, as the number is the mathematical exponent of that power of 100 which expresses the degree of dilution.

in the consecutive complaints. In the latter, aconite, belladonna, and rhus, may become prominent; yet they are seldom useful in the former.

Those who are hardly weaned from red tinctures, may prefer much lower attenuations. If in the above list, some should substitute the 3d or 6th, for the 12th, and the 12th for the 30th, they can be pretty successful, but not as successful as by adhering to the above potencies. Much less can they succeed, if they resort to the hazardous experiment of employing crude drugs in this malady. If the author were charged with the duty of testing the relative merits of the Homœopathic and Allœopathic laws of cure, before an intelligent and impartial tribunal of either school, and if his life depended upon obtaining a verdict in favor of Homœopathy, he would not only select violent and rapid diseases, in preference to such as are mild and chronic, but would administer attenuated medicines, in small doses.

New-York, March 19th, 1849.

Since the first edition of this book was published, the value of the course which it recommends has been extensively tested, in cases of Cholerina and fully-developed Cholera. The Homœopathic practice has been eminently successful during this epidemic, in New York, New Orleans and Cincinnati. When the official statistics shall appear, they will exhibit the same contrast between the results of the Homœopathic and Allœopathic treatment, as in other countries, provided pure Homœopathy is rigidly adhered to by the practitioners of our school.

New York, June 16th, 1849.

CHAPTER 1.

NATURE AND PATHOLOGY OF THE CHOLERA,

WITH REFERENCE TO THE DARK COLOR OF THE BLOOD AND THE DEFICIENCY OF ANIMAL HEAT.

CHARACTERISTICS.

The disease which is now generally known by the name of Cholera, or The Cholera, and which has been denominated Epidemic, Asiatic, Spasmodic and Pestilential Cholera, and Cholera Asphyctica or Asphyxia, agrees in but few particulars with the ordinary Sporadic or Bilious Cholera, known by the name of Cholera Morbus. It usually differs from the latter in the whitish appearance of the alvine evacuations; in the absence of bile in them and in the matters vomited; and the suppression of other secretions, especially that of the urine; in the greater liability to cramps and other spasms; in the coldness of the body, including surface, tongue, breath, &c.; in the livid color of the skin; in the early cessation of the pulse; and in the great rapidity and fatality of the disease.

Dissections reveal but few and slight traces of inflammation or other morbid changes in the solid constituents of the bodies of persons who have died of this disease—none that are constant, and in many cases none at all.

Hence the disease is calculated to confute the theory and paralyze the exertions of the anatomical sect. It is found no less puzzling and intractable by the chemical and mechanical sects; although they have given some attention to the blood, the part in which the most important morbid alterations are found. The chemical Allœopathists have endeavored to supply the deficiency of its salts by artificially introducing them, either by the mouth or the veins; whilst the mechanical Allœopathists, supposing that the thickening of the blood was merely a consequence of the discharge of its watery parts into the intestines, strive to arrest this discharge by opiates and astringents. The most pure and perfect specimen of this practice, is a plan proposed by an Allœopathic medical professor: viz., to cork up the anus.

The hints I have to offer on the pathology of this disease may be of some use, if they serve no other purpose but to dissuade from such mechanical views, and teach that no reliance can be placed on any treatment but that which is specific in its nature and symptomatic in its rule, and which, under the guidance of an unerring law, strikes at the secret springs of morbid action. A consideration of the true source of animal heat will show the futility of all attempts to restore it by hot baths or hot drinks, whilst the vital and chemical processes on which it depends continue to be interrupted—to say nothing of the delusive analogy between actual warmth and that sensation of warmth which is produced by stimulants, and which has led some to attach some importance to these in Cholera.

Another object will be, to point out such relations between certain pathological and ætiological facts, as will afford some clue to the apparently anomalous character of the predisposing causes, to impress the importance of certain precautionary measures relating to diet and regimen, and afford aid in prognosticating the progress of the epidemic.

One of the most remarkable features of *Cholera* in an advanced stage, and of the more perfect types of the disease almost immediately after its onset, is the rapid failure of *animal heat.* The temperature of the whole body is greatly reduced, and some parts acquire a marbly coldness long before death. The coldness of the skin, tongue, breath, &c., I have frequently observed, and others have a thousand times described. These phenomena must be attributed to some impression which the poison—probably introduced through the lungs into the blood—has made upon the nervous system; an impression which interferes with the introduction of oxygen into the blood, or with its chemical action on the carbon and hydrogen.

PHYSIOLOGY OF RESPIRATION

With respect to *animal heat in genera l* the results of Mr. Brodie's experiments were, for a while, thought by many to be fatal to every modification of the chemical theory, from those of Black and Lavoisier to that of Crawford. But the later and more careful experiments and more correct reasonings of Drs. Philip, Legallois, Edwards, and Liebig, have tended to restore the chemical theory, so far at least as it respects the general doctrine of the dependence of calorification on the absorption of oxygen and the production of carbonic acid. But although respiration must be considered essential to animal heat, some physiologists are still disposed to attribute calorification, in part, to the direct actions of the nervous and circulatory systems. The influence of these, however, appears to be indirect. The contact and combination of the oxygen with the blood, is promoted by innervation and circulation, whilst the latter diffuses through the system that caloric, which by the union of oxygen with carbon and hydrogen, is evolved on the same principle as in combustion.

Without dwelling upon the analogy between respiration and combustion, or upon the influence of hydrogen, it will be sufficient barely to allude to a few of the numerous experiments and observations, which prove a necessary *relation* between the amount of *carbonic acid* produced during respiration and that of *caloric* evolved in the system. For example, Legallois effected a diminution in both, by placing an animal in such a position as constrained its respiration. Edwards ascertained that both were affected in a corresponding manner by the influence of the seasons: for in summer, less carbonic acid was formed, and likewise less heat was evolved. The latter fact was not a mere inference from the former, but was established by exposing the same kind of animal to the same freezing mixture in winter and in summer, and finding that in the latter season, the reduction of its temperature was, in a given time, six or eight times as great as in winter.

The *final cause* of this correspondence between the oxygen consumed and the temperature of the surrounding medium, is as obvious as it is interesting. This is a beneficent provision, by which, as well as by a variable cutaneous and pulmonary transpiration, the Author of nature has, in some degree, defended man and the inferior animals against the vicissitudes of the seasons. But neither our limits nor the nature of our subject will allow us to dwell upon this interesting topic.

That correspondence between the degrees of aeration and those of animal heat, which has been already alluded to, *extends to the whole animal kingdom.* It will be found to exist, whether we compare the warm-blooded animals with those called cold-blooded, or the different species of either of these grand divisions with each other. The respiration of the lower orders of animals is, however, so imperfect, and their temperature is, consequently, so little elevated above that of the media in which they reside, that the evidence of the extension of the above law to them was at one time merely analogical. But discoveries in electro-magnetism have suggested an extremely delicate thermometer, by means of which, the relation, that in the higher classes of animals, is known to exist between animal heat and aeration, is proved to hold even among different species of insects as compared with each other; those which produce more carbonic acid, possess a more elevated temperature. This may therefore be regarded as a universal law.

There is no difficulty in understanding why the skin should have a dark color, whenever the deficiency of animal heat in the body, and of the oxygen used and the carbonic acid formed during respiration, evince an accumulation of carbon in the blood.

APPLICATION TO THE PATHOLOGY OF CHOLERA.

That *a dark color of the blood is one of the characteristics of Cholera*, is well known. To this color of the blood we are to attribute the livid color of the surface of the body—a color which is not, however, identical with that of the blood, but depends partly upon the color of the medium through which the blood is seen.

In this disease, there is frequently no sensible difference between the color of the venous and that of the arterial blood. Many physicians have compared the blood to tar or treacle. The blood drawn from a patient was found by Dr. Reid Clanny to be as black as tar, and to contain more than twice as much carbon as healthy blood. It was tasteless, and contained no carbonic acid or gas of any kind. The want of taste cannot be wholly referred to the elimination of salts, but affords evidence of a defect in the respiratory function; for the stronger taste is one of the properties acquired by this liquid in traversing the lungs; and as superior sapidity distinguishes arterial from venous blood, we might naturally expect it to distinguish venous blood from supervenous.

Whether the carbon which he obtained by his ultimate analysis, previously existed in a free state, as he, in my opinion, too hastily concluded, is of little consequence. None of those who have objected to his views, have produced any ultimate analysis which militates against his conclusion, that there is a great excess of carbon, compared with that which exists in normal blood. In the controversy which has been carried on by Dr. Clanny and others, the object has been, either to prove or disprove the existence of carbon in the blood in a *free* state, and the excess of *uncombined* carbon in cholera blood. The decision of this point is probably of little importance in the pathology of Cholera; at any rate, it does not, in the least, affect the question which I am considering. The manner in which the elements of that part of the coloring matter which contains carbon, are arranged, whether in binary, ternary or quaternary combination, has never been determined; but Brande, Engelhart and Michaelis have shown that the coloring matter of the blood consists of an animal matter, associated with a minute quantity of iron and some earthy salts; and this animal matter, of which the coloring matter appears chiefly to consist, was found by Michaelis to contain more than fifty-three per cent. of carbon. Now in what degree the carbon of the coloring matter may vary in different kinds of blood, I find no satisfactory data for determining. The furnishing of these is, perhaps, a service which pathology has yet to expect from chemistry. But even conceding, that a given quantity of the coloring matter of cholera blood, contains only the same amount of carbon as the same quantity of the coloring matter of normal blood, (and no one has pretended that it contains less,) it can, I think, be shown, that the whole amount of carbon in the coloring matter of the former, far exceeds the whole amount in the coloring matter of the latter. For according to the researches of Dr. Thompson, professor of chemistry in Glasgow, the coloring matter of cholera blood, as deduced from the mean of his results, is "little short of *four times* the quantity of coloring matter of healthy blood." Dr. Clanny's *proximate* analysis afforded nearly the same result. This may be reconciled with the result of his *destructive* distillation in another instance, in which he obtained only about twice as much carbon from cholera blood as from healthy blood, by considering that both fibrine and albumen contain rather more than fifty per cent. of carbon, and that the great increase of coloring matter, is partly compensated by the diminution of the sum of these other carbonaceous principles. That this will explain the apparent discrepancy, might be shown by the numerical results. But that the change in the absolute amount of fibrine is small, compared with that of the coloring matter, is evident from Dr. Thompson's testimony, that the fibrine and coloring matter of healthy blood added together, amount to less than one-half the coloring matter in cholera blood. Notwithstanding all that has been said by the opponents of hyperanthraxis, I am unable to discern, why the quantities of carbon obtained from two portions of blood, submitted under the same circumstances, to destructive distillation in a close vessel, may not correctly show the relative proportions that actually existed in them. The only sound objection refers to the *state* in which the carbon existed.

Now, that this vast accumulation of carbon in the blood of a cholera patient is absolute, and not merely a relative increase, resulting from incrassation, in consequence of the removal of its aqueous portion, by profuse evacuations or any other cause, we may readily convince ourselves from a comparison of the numerical results in Dr. Thompson's table, by which it will be found, that the proportional diminution of water in cholera blood is very small, compared either with the proportional increase of coloring matter as shown by his experiments, or of carbon as shown by Dr. Clanny's. How then can it be true, that the addition of the dejections to the blood would restore it to its normal condition? Are not even Dr. O'Shaugnessy's results with respect to the albumen, opposed to the above conclusion which has been drawn from his analysis? The *history* of this epidemic is opposed to it. It has been long since and repeatedly observed, by those who have been familiar with the disease in its most malignant and perfect form, that the most rapid and intractable cases were generally attended with slight, if any, alvine evacuations. Not to cite other authorities, Mr.

Orton, at Bombay, and other surgeons in that vicinity, stated that in many cases there was no purging, in some no vomiting, and in others neither, and that these were by far the most dangerous cases, and that the patients died under them, often in an hour or two; and that, without spasms and with scarcely any vomiting or purging, all the secretions appeared to be in many cases entirely suspended.* Conceding the possibility, that in some cases, the contents of the alimentary canal may not have been examined, still, from what we know of its dimensions, and from the effects of equivalent evacuations in other diseases, a theory which can be defended only by a supposed accumulation in such cases, must be considered untenable. Has it not been chiefly in those places which have been but slightly visited, that we find pathologists disposed to found a theory on profuse evacuations? Under such circumstances, these may perhaps merit all the attention which has been bestowed upon them; although the most fatal alterations of the blood, and the suppression of urine and other secretions, must often, if not always, depend upon another cause.†

* Good's Study of Med. I. 178.

† There is little doubt that the secretion of urine may be both increased and diminished, by some agencies which have no direct influence on the action of the kidneys, or

It is hardly necessary to remark, that the presence of an immense excess of carbon in the blood, manifests a defect in the decarbonizing process of the system. It may be less obvious, though hardly less certain, that the observed *absence of carbonic acid* in the blood, in this disease, depends upon a similar cause. A considerable quantity of this gas exists in healthy blood; and it might be asked, why the same cause, from which, in this disease, the blood retains its carbon, does not also make it retain the carbonic acid. I answer, it is because the carbonic acid eliminated during respiration, derives its oxygen from the inspired air; and when little or no oxygen is absorbed, we should expect little or no carbonic acid to be formed. From the absence or deficiency of carbonic acid, I should infer, that in this disease, there exists *more difficulty in obtaining the advantages of in-*

the quantity of serum in the blood. Even Dr. Cullen acknowledged his suspicion of this, opposed as it was to his favorite theory. His modesty and candor are worthy of the imitation of those who are ambitious of framing *complete* theories in medicine. He says, that "besides the increased quantity of water in the mass of the blood, or a stimulus particularly applied to the kidneys, there may be a medicine which, by a general operation on the system, may promote the secretion of urine.—My candor obliges me to mention this; but I do not find myself at present in a condition to prosecute the inquiry.—Materia Med. vol. II. p. 556.

spiration than those of expiration—in forming carbonic acid than in eliminating it.

In the phenomena presented after death, there are many striking coincidences between Cholera and asphyxia from other causes; the same fluidity of the blood, for hours after death, the same tendency of the body after death to an increase of warmth and diminution of lividity, as in cases where the respiration is suspended by hanging or drowning, or not established by a closure of the foramen ovale. I have known these phenomena to be presented after death in the case of a premature child, which was born at the end of the 7th month, and lived till the fourth day after its birth; and I have observed some of them in cases of death by hanging and drowning, and I believe them to be characteristic of asphyxia. They frequently inspire the friends of the deceased with the vain hope of effecting a resuscitation.

The following case will illustrate some of the foregoing remarks, as well as the effect produced on the blood by certain salts, which, since the experiments of Dr. Stevens, have been supposed to perform an important part in the function of respiration. A son of Mr. V. V., ætat. eighteen months, had fallen into a cistern of water, and lain, as was supposed, a quarter of an hour or more, and had been taken out about half an hour before my arrival. We attempted to re-establish respiration, by inflating the lungs, not only by the mouth, but by a pair of bellows fitted to a flexible tube which was introduced into the trachea. Other means were used, but to no effect. About two hours after the death of the child, the jugular vein was opened. A dark-colored blood ran freely. Three or four ounces were taken. Its coagulability was so slight, that it required a plaster to arrest it. As the plasticity or coagulability of arterial blood as compared with venous, is a property acquired by respiration, it might be expected, that the supervenous blood of Cholera and other species of asphyxia, would be more deficient in this property than ordinary venous blood. And such is the fact. In the above case, it coagulated very slowly and imperfectly after its removal from the vein, resembling, in this respect, the blood drawn during life from Cholera patients. After half an hour had elapsed, about one-third of it had not coagulated, although the temperature of the air was about 70°. The upper part, which had been exposed to the air, was coagulated to a certain depth, and its color at the surface had become rather brighter. On inclining the vessel, the dark, thick and uncoagulated fluid broke through the coagulated crust, and flowed sluggishly across it, presenting an appearance somewhat similar to that of Cholera blood, which from its consistence and blackness, has so often been compared to molasses and tar. The parts of the coagulum below the surface were also dark-colored. It appeared evident, that air favored coagulation, and was more essential to the production of the florid color, but did not appear to effect the latter as readily and perfectly as in the case of normal or healthy blood. Muriate of soda was then added to one portion, and carbonate of soda to another. The latter had a marked effect, rendering it florid. This experiment, and others made on normal venous blood, have convinced me that it is unphilosophical to infer from the effect of salts in reddening cholera blood, that the asphyxia which produces its dark color depends on the deficiency of saline ingredients in the blood, even though such deficiency should by analysis be shown to exist; for in the case above mentioned, and in others alluded to, a similar change of color was produced by the salts, although there was no reason to suspect any greater deficiency of saline ingredients than ordinarily exists in venous blood. The circumstance that the color of the blood was less influenced by exposure to air than ordinary venous blood, shows that a defect in this property is not peculiar to Cholera, nor to disease of any kind, properly so called, but appears to be characteristic of asphyxia in general, whether induced by disease or suddenly caused by interrupting the respiration of an individual previously in health, when there have been no intestinal discharges to drain the salts from the system.

I consider the defect in coagulability as also common to all those cases where a want of due oxygenation is the sole or chief cause of death. Excessive exercise and violent mental emotions, when they occur suddenly, are said to produce this state of the blood; and it appears to me an interesting fact, that these are also among the causes which tend to prevent its oxygenation. Another correspondence not less curious is, that in the fœtus, whose respiration has never been established, the venous and arterial blood, like that of the victims of Cholera, is nearly identical; the blood is not coagulable, has an unctuous feel, and does not take the vermilion color on exposure to the air; and according to Fourcroy, it has its coloring matter darker and more abundant, and contains no fibrine. It therefore remarkably resembles Cholera blood. Would it not seem, from these facts and considerations, that the coagulation of the fibrine, and even its existence as such, are more dependent on respiration than has been hitherto suspected; and that the deficiency of this principle, as well as the existence of most of the other peculiarities which distinguish cholera blood from normal blood, result chiefly from its defective aeration, and are what might be expected in asphyxia from any other cause? Dr. Good admits the want of coagulability of the blood in cases of electrical, and Broussais in cases of gaseous asphyxia. Combining these two authorities, relating respectively to asphyxia caused by lightning and that caused by the irrespirable and deleterious gases, with my own observations on other varieties of asphyxia, I am led to infer the generality of the above law. That the tarry appearance of cholera blood results from want of aeration, is also confirmed by the fact, that the same appearance may be immediately produced by prussic acid, but never unless given in such doses as to occasion difficulty of breathing.*

* Am. Jour. of Med. Sci. vol. xi. p. 501, from an European Journal.—Dr. Hartwig, who made this discovery, blackened the blood by different acids, but could not, it appears, produce this effect by *nitric* acid.—Ibid. I have, however, ascertained by experiment, that nitric acid *does* render the sanguineous coloring matter black as seen by *reflected* (though not as seen by transmitted) light. Has this distinction between the reflected and transmitted light been made by those who have experimented on the blood? By other experiments on blood more nearly normal, I have proved, that the effect of saline substances on the blood at one temperature, cannot be inferred from experi-

A defect in calorification and sanguification may exist, in a slight degree, in an early stage of the disease, and not become the most obvious characteristic till the last. Before any profuse alvine evacuations had taken place, I have, in several instances, observed a coldness of the hands and feet, a blueness of the under eyelid, and a preternaturally dark color of the blood drawn from the arm. In this stage also, Dr. Baird found the heat of the skin below the healthy standard. Dr. McIntyre notices a slightly discolored state of the under eyelid, as among the most frequent premonitory symptoms. Others have observed, that the dark color of the skin frequently prevails as a premonitory symptom from one to ten days, whilst there is no peculiarity in the evacuations.

That no other disease effects so remarkable a change in the composition, color and temperature of the blood, must be admitted; also that these alterations are disproportionate to the amount of alvine evacuations, whether we compare different

ments made at another; and that the blackening of crassamentum by hot water, is not—as has been asserted—dependent on the extraction of its saline matters; and also, that the change of color produced in the sanguineous coloring matter by heat, is not the result of the extrication of oxygen or any other gas. For these experiments, vide Transactions of the Medical Society of the State of New-York, vol. ii. p. 181.

cases of this disease, or this disease with others; although, neither the physiology of respiration, the chemistry of normal blood, nor the chemical pathology of Cholera, is so complete, as to justify any positive opinion as to the precise time, nor any complete theory of the manner, in which these changes commence. Indeed, the pathogeny of most diseases is obscure; and pathology seldom detects the first links in the chain of morbid phenomena. In Cholera, it can hardly be considered more fortunate with respect to some of the subsequent ones. There is no complete theory; and I do not offer the above as such.

Fortunately for mankind, Hahnemann has discovered a law of cure which is not based upon pathological speculations. The want of such a law and of any reliable guide, is the real cause of the want of unanimity and I may say the uncertainty, confusion and anarchy, that prevails in the alloeopathic school. These have, in the case of no disease, been more conspicuous than in relation to Cholera, and never more so than at the present time.

CHAPTER II.

ÆTIOLOGY,

ESPECIALLY WITH REFERENCE TO THE PREDISPOSING AND OCCASIONAL CAUSES.

PRELIMINARY ÆTIOLOGICAL REMARKS.

The peculiar cause of the Cholera is unknown. Hahnemann, and some other learned men, have thought it to be probably an animated miasm. It seems frequently to manifest some self-moving power, or at least to be capable of diffusing itself and of travelling, independently of transportation by human beings, or by the wind. Whatever be its nature, whether animalcular, gaseous, or electrical, it must possess extreme tenuity to escape detection; and its terrific potency is well calculated to rebuke the scepticism of those who sneer at the evidence of efficiency in attenuated medicines, and in everything not cognizable by their senses of sight, smell, hearing, taste or touch.

But as the nature of the cause of Cholera is involved in obscurity, and as I shall under the head of infection, give some views in relation to its propagation, I shall here limit myself to its *predisposing* and *occasional causes*, as related to the pathological phenomena above considered.

If we say that Cholera is attended with great depression of the vital forces, and that the predisposing causes are such as depress these forces or produce general debility, we make a statement which is, to a certain extent and in a certain sense, correct. but is deficient in definite meaning, and but partially true in any sense. If it were strictly and generally true, we should expect that individuals who were robust and muscular, and at the middle period of life, would, cæteris paribus, have a comparative immunity from the disease. But this is far from being the fact. The views about to be presented, not only refer to a definite function, but to a class of correspondences which are more marked in Cholera than in any other disease.

There are many reasons for believing, that during the prevalence of Cholera there is some wide-spread miasm or other aerial epidemic influence tending to diminish the aeration of the blood. We have perhaps some indirect evidence, in the nearly simultaneous prevalence of certain diseases in which the blood is similarly affected, though in an inferior degree. Is there not in many places, either antecedently, or subsequently, an increased prevalence of certain diseases which are attended with dark blood, such as measles, and typhus and other malignant and occasionally anomalous fevers? For weeks and months before the acknowledged incursion of Cholera, there are frequently cases of disease which in these respects nearly resemble it, as I am convinced by my own observations and those of many other physicians.

But to give more satisfactory proof of this connexion between Cholera and respiration, I shall proceed to examine, whether the history of Cholera does not present a class of etiological facts, which, considered in connexion with the results of experiments that have been made on respiration, without any reference to Cholera, tend to confirm the foregoing views with regard to one of its principal if not essential features.

ATMOSPHERIC HEAT.

The influence of external *heat* on respiration was discovered by Crawford. His experiments and those of others have satisfactorily shown, that the quantity of oxygen consumed and of carbonic acid produced during respiration, is less as the temperature of the air is more elevated. All who have experimented on the subject, with but one exception, have detected this influence of temperature. Crawford found that a Guinea pig, confined in air at the temperature of 55° Fah., consumed double the quantity of oxygen which it did in air at 104°. In the case of human respiration, Lavoisier and Seguin ascertained, that the quantity at 57° is to that at 82° as 1344 is to 1210. Delaroche, in his last series of experiments, made the average ratio about as six to five at the temperatures tried by him. He found, that by elevation of temperature, the production of carbonic acid was diminished, and the absorption of oxygen diminished in a still higher ratio. More recently Dr. Edwards has examined the effect of different seasons, and found that the *long-continued* actions of heat and cold affect the respiration as a vital function; the oxygen consumed being less in summer, even when the air in which the animal is confined at the time, is of the same density and temperature. Moreover, from the experiments above related respecting the influence of sudden changes of temperature, as well as from the known effect of temperature on density, it appears to me evident, that its physical changes between winter and summer, must be such as to make the immediate influence of heat conspire with its gradual physiological effects, and render the consumption in winter and summer still more disproportionate. The influence of heat in diminishing the consumption of oxygen may be considered as established.

On the other hand, few facts are better established, than the influence of hot climates and the warm season of the year of predisposing to Cholera. The epidemic in 1817—which subsequently spread over a considerable portion of the globe, and arrived here in 1832—commenced in summer in the hot climate of Hindostan; it has generally, in all climates, been much checked if not extinguished by winter; also on cold, elevated mountains. Its ravages in Mexico proved, that it can rise to a great height above the surface of the sea in *warm* climates. In Russia, the southern regions were those where it spread most widely and rapidly; and those towns which it entered at the end of autumn, suffered but slightly.* It is no evidence against these views, that it lingered in winter, in some of the highly-heated, ill-ventilated and filthy rooms of that country. Even in Persia and Asia Minor, the influence of winter on epidemic cholera was manifest during several successive years.† This influence of temperature has been confirmed by the progress of the disease on the western continent. In 1832, it commenced in spring, and until the autumnal cold, nothing impeded its rapid march or changed its malignant character. Both were restored by the heat of the ensuing spring; and again suspended by winter. In its present second tour, the influence of temperature has been manifest. At the Quarantine on Staten Island, it disappeared at the commencement of the first severe cold of January; and even the cold of December was sufficient to arrest it in the city of New-York, which had been slightly inoculated. We owe our present immunity, our respite, to cold. The recent epidemic in New-Orleans, prevailed in its greatest intensity when the thermometer stood on its greatest height, and disappeared when the weather became sufficiently cold.

* Report of M. Moreau de Jonnes.

† Report of the French Academy.

BECOMING CHILLED BY COLD AIR OR BY COLD BATHING.

It is remarkable, that the transient application of a cold sufficient to produce a certain degree of *chilliness*, produces the same effect as long-continued heat, both in relation to Cholera and to respiration.

It is known that becoming chilled greatly increases the liability to Cholera.

Dr. Edwards found that in the animals on which he experimented, as well as in man, the becoming chilled, effected more than a mere transient reduction of temperature; it actually weakened the heat-producing power. This was proved by its requiring a longer time for the animal to recover its warmth after the second exposure than after the first. He states also, that in a severe winter, in which the Seine was frozen, a young man in attempting to cross it, broke the ice and fell into the water; but being strong and active, he succeeded in getting out. His health did not suffer; but for three days he had a continual sensation of cold. This was not so simple an affection of the nervous system as a mere prolongation of a strong impression, but it was an alteration of function—a diminution of the heat-producing power. *

* Vide—Influence of Physical Agents on Life, by W. F. Edwards, M. D., F. R. S.

We hardly need refer to such high authority for facts like this last. Most persons are conscious, after being excessively chilled and then warmed by the heat of a fire, that on returning immediately into the cold air, they for a while experience more chilliness than at the first period of the previous exposure. It is unphilosophical to refer these first effects of being chilled (or taking cold) to check of perspiration; for perspiration, as connected with the evaporation which attends it, is physically a cooling process; and the check of it would immediately produce warmth, were it not for the operation of the principle above stated.

It is well to add here a word of *application*, at a time when many exaggerate the advantages, and overlook the dangers, of powerful *baths*. This delusion will have its victims, especially during the prevalence of Cholera. Cleanliness may, and it should be preserved, without making any strong or durable impression, either of heat or cold. This is the true criterion of safe ablution. In addition to the danger of excessive bathing to the community in general, there is one which should not be overlooked by those who are under Homœopathic treatment, either for the cure of disease or for preparing their systems to resist the epidemic. Strongly-impressing baths disturb the action of remedies. Hahnemann justly considered their present effect as analogous to that of large doses of drugs, and their frequent repetition, as tending to retard the cure of chronic diseases. I shall, under another head, give some rules for bathing, but at present advert to other predisposing causes of Cholera.

THE NIGHT SEASON.

It has been ascertained, that the quantity of carbonic acid produced, is less in the *night* than in the day-time. Whether this depends directly on the absence of the sun or not, is not certainly known. From the well established relation between the aeration of the blood and animal heat, considered in connexion with the opinion which Dr. Edwards' experiments led him to entertain, that there is less animal heat evolved during sleep, we may conclude that sleep contributes in some measure to the defect of aeration. Rest may be added, as *moderate* exercise increases oxygenation. But this has no material influence on the value of the above-mentioned fact, except that it tends to confirm the influence of night, the usual season of rest and of sleep. Now it has been frequently stated, that the attacks

4*

of Cholera are generally more frequent during the night. At Smyrna, in October, 1831, and in some other places, the mortality, it was said, occurred principally in the night. The French Royal Academy of Medicine stated in their report that the invasion of the disease had generally taken place in the night and toward morning. Now Dr. Prout found that the carbonic acid in the respired air, reached its minimum at half past eight in the evening, and remained at the minimum state till half past three in the morning. As the effects of this defective aeration of the blood, are accumulating during the whole of this period during which it remains at the minimum state, should we not expect that, in proportion as the influence of night predominated among the causes of the disease, it would manifest itself oftener towards morning? And is not the principle analogous to that on which depend the more wide and rapid extension and the increased severity of Cholera and some other malignant diseases which are connected, though less remarkably, with a defective aeration of the blood, at the close of that season of the year in which this function is at its minimum? A similar principle is applied in physics, to the explanation of the observed time of maximum temperature both of the day and year.

DEPRESSING PASSIONS, FATIGUE, FASTING, AND ALCOHOL.

Dr. Prout ascertained, by direct experiment, that the quantity of carbonic acid produced during respiration is diminished by the *depressing passions*, or even *strong* mental *emotions* of any kind; by *long-continued and violent exercise*; by *fasting*; and by *intemperate habits*, and even the *moderate use of alcoholic liquors*. It is well known, that all these are powerful predisposing causes of epidemic *Cholera*. The disease has been frequently favored by the fatiguing marches of armies and the privations which they have suffered; by the existence of poverty with its attendant evils of excessive labor and scanty food; by violent anger, by the depressing passions, such as the fear of the disease itself; and by intemperate habits, and even the moderate use of alcoholic liquors. The want of success which has generally attended the administration of alcohol in this disease would not of itself be conclusive, but it may have some weight. The foregoing views respecting the causes and nature of epidemic Cholera, and a knowledge of the specific action of alcohol in diminishing the oxygenation of the blood, in all individuals, however temperate and healthy, might have led us to anticipate that its influence in predisposing to this disease, would not be confined to the broken-down drunkard. This inference from theory is confirmed by experience. In relation to that form of the disease, in which at the height of the epidemic in Vienna, it most nearly approximated to the perfect type, and in which the seizure was sudden, the evacuations almost or altogether wanting, the cramps severe, and the fatal termination in most cases in a few hours, it was observed that a middle age, vigor of constitution, and such a use of gin as had not materially affected it, were predisposing causes.* The last is a practice which diminishes the aeration of the blood, and the two former are circumstances under which, as has often been shown, such diminution can be tolerated with least impunity. In relation to ardent spirits, as predisposing to this disease, mistakes have arisen from too wide a distinction between *drinking* and *drunkenness*. These mistakes would be corrected by physiological views.

ABSTINENCE FROM ANIMAL FOOD.

Dr. Fyfe proved by experiment, that the carbonic acid was *reduced to nearly one*

* Lond. Lancet for June 23d, 1832.

half by vegetable diet. Now this is the diet which has predominated in those countries, in those cities and in those classes of society, in which the disease has been most fatal, whether in Asia, Europe or America. It is true, some physicians have recommended vegetable food during the epidemic, interdicting only unripe vegetables, and a few kinds generally admitted to be peculiarly unwholesome. But this preference for vegetable food must proceed rather from an incorrect theory, and from their experience in other diseases supposed by them to be analogous, than from their experience or that of the world in this disease.* In the report published by the authority of the French Academy, it is affirmed, that during the Cholera at Calcutta, "those who lived on vegetable substances were first taken off; and that women and children seemed to be spared." I quote the whole passage, as the latter part affords some evidence, that this influence of vegetable food is not, as some have supposed, referrible merely to the debility and consequent irritability induced by it.

Moreover, that it was mode of living,

* Most species of *grain*, however, being more easy of digestion and containing more azote than most other parts of vegetables, make a nearer approximation to animal food, and are hence less injurious than some other vegetable substances.

and not idiosyncrasy, that rendered the Hindoos so much more liable to the disease than the English residents, may be argued from the fact, that the native soldiers, whose mode of living was more similar to that of the English, enjoyed a similar degree of exemption. Indeed, it was every where observed, that those who subsisted on vegetable food, were selected as the first victims. Perhaps it may be worthy of remark, that the unusual mortality in Paris, where at the least twenty thousand of the inhabitants were carried off in a month, occurred during the season of Lent. Immediately after Easter the virulence of the disease rapidly abated. The proportion of vegetable food is usually great among a French population. May not the severe Cholera of Montreal and New Orleans in 1832, be cited as in some degree examples of its influence? On the ensuing spring, the disease, after its winter's sleep, awoke in the Catholic city of Havana, in the season of Lent. It numbered among its victims many of the most respectable and religious citizens, and produced a mortality unprecedented in the history of its ravages in the western hemisphere.* Were

* Among other respectable individuals who fell victims, was the Arshbishop of Havana. On some days 900 are said to have died out of a population of about 180,000. Not having access, however, to official documents, I extract

these isolated facts, they would merit less regard. But the influence of vegetable food has been generally observed to predispose to Cholera, and even to epizootics strongly resembling it; but never, in any instance which I have heard, among animals exclusively carnivorous. I need only allude to the epizootic which prevailed among several species of herbivorous ani-

this from the newspapers, as also the following account of the recommencement of the march of the disease in Louisiana, nearly at the same time. The following is from the Albany Argus of April 15th, 1833. "The Louisiana Republican, printed at Franklin, in the Attakapas region, says that the Cholera has begun to assume, in that quarter, a more formidable appearance. At first, few cases proved fatal, except those which occurred among the colored population; persons of temperate habits were seldom attacked." [This shows the influence of alcohol.] "But of late, citizens *particularly noted* for their temperance have fallen victims." [This shows, perhaps, the combined effect of heat, vegetable diet, and fasting.] The St. Martinsville (Lou.) Courier of 22d March, gives a similar account of its prevalence in that place and its vicinity. "As it was nearly stationary during the winter, we thought that the salubrity of our situation would preserve us; but within the last three weeks, it appears to have extended its exterminating influence, and we have already to deplore the loss of several respectable inhabitants of our parish, as also a great number of slaves." Now it is worthy of notice, that the 24th of Feb. was the first Sunday in Lent; and it would seem that the extension of its "exterminating influence" commenced about a week afterwards. What intemperance did for the lower and dissolute, did not fasting and vegetable diet contribute to effect for the higher and religious classes? Those who are better acquainted with their habits can judge.

mals in Scotland, and to the mortality among the fowls of Choisi near Paris; to their white alvine discharges; and the dark color assumed by their combs, affording, from their translucence, an index to the color of the blood.

From the effects of vegetable diet and abstinence from food, I must believe, that a fast in either of these senses, during the epidemic, would tend to aggravate the awful calamity which it might be proposed for the purpose of averting; yet, on the other hand, as strong emotions, and especially the depressing passions, have been shown to produce an influence similar to that of fasting, it is evident that a religious frame of mind, a calm and cheerful reliance on Divine Providence, must be among the best preservatives. During the prevalence of Cholera, it should be considered a sacred duty to avoid fasting, except so far as fasting is dictated by want of appetite.

OPPRESSION OF THE DIGESTIVE ORGANS, WITH FOOD INDIGESTIBLE IN QUALITY OR EXCESSIVE IN QUANTITY.

This is another cause of impaired calorific function, as well as of Cholera. During the first stage of a digestion rendered laborious by indigestible food or over-eating, all persons—especially those of weak digestive powers—are conscious of some degree of chilliness on exposure to cold. This, as Dr. Edwards has explained in the cases before cited, is not merely a simple nervous impression, but an alteration of function, a diminution of the power of generating animal heat.

Now it is known, that excess in eating, even in the case of wholesome food, and the use of indigestible substances, as crude and flatulent vegetables, clams, the meat of young animals, &c., especially by persons of weak digestion, frequently disposes to an attack of Cholera.

CROWDED OR INSUFFICIENTLY VENTILATED ROOMS.

The *air* of *rooms* which are occupied by too many persons, or insufficiently ventilated, diminishes the aeration of the blood and the generation of animal heat, and also predisposes to an attack of Cholera. It is unnecessary to cite any proofs of the former proposition. Air deficient in oxygen and charged with carbonic acid, cannot properly sustain the calorific function. Its effect in predisposing to Cholera, the history of this epidemic sufficiently manifests. The principle here referred to, is distinct from that of infection. When the disease has once entered a room, both principles cooperate. But crowded and ill-ventilated rooms not only conduce to the communication of the disease when once admitted, but they invite it to enter.

The occupants of basements seem, cæteris paribus, to be more liable to the disease. This may be owing to the combined effect of carbonic acid and humidity, and perhaps of the tendency of Cholera miasm to travel into low places. That some of the other circumstances above enumerated, exert on the miasm a physical influence, which conspires with their physiological influence on man, in exciting the disease, is not improbable.

NEGLECT OF PERSONAL CLEANLINESS.

The accumulation of cutaneous filth sustains to respiration, animal heat and the state of the blood, and to Cholera, a relation similar to that of the ten other circumstances above considered: but its influence is less striking. By mechanically obstructing the cutaneous pores, filth must in some measure diminish the aeration of the blood, which is known to be effected in part by the skin. There is here, as in the lungs, an absorption of oxygen and elimination of carbonic acid. There is in man, a cutaneous as well as pulmonary respiration; though it is less remarkable than in frogs and other animals of the order batrachia, which will survive the loss of their lungs longer than that of their skin.

But in man, the obstruction of the cutaneous pores is more important in its relation to the pulmonary than to the cutaneous respiration, or even to the cutaneous perspiration; as was intimated when treating of the effects of being chilled. The liquid transpired could, if suppressed, be chiefly eliminated by the kidneys; but although other evils would ultimately result from this retention, the first morbid effects of obstructing the cutaneous pores—even as it relates to transpiration—seem to relate chiefly to the oxygenating and calorific function.

UNGENERALIZED FACTS.

Among the circumstances which physiologists have found to diminish the quantity of oxygen, there are, in addition to those which have been enumerated, a few others, the influence of which in predisposing to this disease requires further investigation. These are the use of tea; the administration of nitric acid; affecting the system by a course of mercury; and placing the body in a posture which impedes respiration. I am acquainted with no general etiological fact in relation to these, which militates against the foregoing views; and from the evidence above adduced, in relation to agencies similar to these in one of their physiological relations, I believe that persons by taking green tea, nitric acid, blue pills or calomel, would be more liable to Cholera.

On the other hand, among the predisposing causes of Cholera, there are some, whose influence on the consumption of oxygen requires further investigation.

Many cases of Asiatic Cholera have been produced by cathartics. I have known several instances. I might give a plausible explanation by which such facts could be brought under the above law; but I prefer abstaining from all hypothesis.

In the same class of ungeneralized facts, I shall for similar reasons, place the influence of certain changes in the hygrometric, barometric and electrical states of the atmosphere. These are so generally connected, that simultaneous and repeated observations, and a nice discrimination, would be requisite to determine their separate influences even on cholera. In August, 1832, I observed at two different times, a considerable *depression* of the barometer and elevation of the dewpoint, and at both times, there was, I believe, a sudden and considerable increase of the disease both in Albany and Schenectady. As the epidemic, having commenced at different times in these two neighboring cities, was not in the same stage, these simultaneous changes must be attributed to a meteorological influence. If humidity was the cause, humidity as detected by the hygrometer, seemed to have more influence than rain. That the effect depended partly on an electrical change preceding a storm, is not improbable. Finally, there are many agents whose influences both on the consumption of oxygen and the production of Cholera are alike unknown. If, as appears from numerous considerations above stated, there is any law connecting these influences, then experiments for determining the effect of these agents on respiration, might lead to important practical applications in relation to the prevention, if not to the treatment of the disease. In applying the results, however, regard should be had to the difference between the immediate and remote effects on respiration ; these are frequently opposite.

RECAPITULATION.

Without the aid of any mere hypothesis, I have shown, that there is a remarkable correspondence between certain classes of physiological and ætiological facts, in relation to the Cholera. This correspondence is interesting on account of the dependence of animal heat and the florid color of arterial blood on respiration, considered in connexion with the fact, that in an advanced state of dangerous cases of every variety of this disease, and in an early stage of the severer varieties, no pathological phenomena are more constant, than a dark color of the blood and a temperature below the normal standard.

As a large proportion of the occasional or predisposing causes are in a great measure under the control of man, a statement of these and of the scientific evidence of their influence, will tend to inspire hope and promote safety.

I have shown that physiology concurs with general experience, in proving the following to be the principal predisposing causes of the Cholera; viz., 1st, *hot climates and hot seasons;* 2d, *becoming chilled by cold air or by cold bathing;* 3d, *the night season;* 4th, *fear and other depressing emotions;* 5th, *violent and excessively fatiguing exercise;* 6th, *total fasting*, i. e. *abstinence* from *all food;* 7th, *partial fasting*, i. e. *abstinence from animal food;* 8th, *oppressing the stomach with food indigestible in quality or excessive in quantity;* 9th, *the moderate as well as intemperate use of alcoholic drinks;* 10th, *crowded or insufficiently ventilated rooms;* and 11th, *neglect of personal cleanliness.*

The order in which these are enumerated, has no reference to their relative potency, but to their natural affinities.

CHAPTER III.

DOCTRINE OF INFECTION

WITH REFERENCE TO THIS DISEASE.

ERROR OF THE PREVALENT DOCTRINE.

An opinion extensively entertained by the profession, is, that there is a certain class of diseases, including small pox, measles, scarlatina and hooping cough, which an individual may take on coming near a patient affected with them, although the intermediate air be pure; and that there is another class of diseases—including plague, yellow fever, typhus fever, dysentery and cholera—which an individual cannot take, unless the intermediate air between him and the patient is impure, and that he takes these from the air, and not by any specific poison derived either directly or indirectly from the patient. The former class of diseases, they denominate contagious; the latter class, infectious.

But in both cases, the disease *is* communicated through the air, and in consequence of its contamination; and in both cases by a specific poison, else the same kind of disease as that with which the first patient was affected would not be reproduced. These classes of disease, when communicated through the air, differ, not in the *principle* or *mode* of communication, but in the quantity or *dose* of the poison, which is requisite for reproducing the disease.

The terms contagion and infection, as now extensively used in a technical sense, serve only to conceal the want of precise ideas, and the defects of a false mode of reasoning. Whence the disputes and hesitation of learned academies—and of the medical world generally—in relation to this subject? In my opinion, this confusion, disagreement and indecision arise from not viewing the subject in a mathematical point of view, that is, in its relation to the science of *quantity*. The popular mind is prone to inquire about the *existence* of certain *things* or entities, rather than their quantitative relations. It asks, is there infection in this disease or in that? It does not think to inquire, whether there is *more* or *less* infecting power. It does not suspect that this is the only difference in many diseases in regard to their power of propagating themselves. The medical mind, perhaps from deficiency of mathematical training, is extensively infected with this same intellectual vice. Physicians, instead of recognizing degrees in the infecting power, generally found their distinctions on modes and media of transmission. Again, instead of recognizing a great diversity, as they would if they had hit on the true principle of distinction, they assume that all except a few diseases are incommunicable under any circumstances; and through those that they acknowledge capable of propagation, they arbitrarily draw a single line, and denominate the whole group on one side of that line contagious, and the whole group on the other side infectious. They have not yet perceived that what they call infection, considered as a property of the disease, is merely the contagious property in less intensity. For convenience, I shall use the terms infection and infectious in their most comprehensive sense, which embraces all modes of communication.

INDEFINITENESS OF THE PROBLEM.

To ask whether Asiatic Cholera is infectious, is like asking whether diluted alcohol is an intoxicating drink. Is diluted alcohol an intoxicating drink, or is it not? Does not every one perceive, that for the solution of this problem, the requisite data are not given in the question? It is indefinite in three respects; viz., first, as to the degree of dilution of the alcohol; secondly, as to the quantity to be taken; and thirdly, as to the susceptibility of the drinker—to its intoxicating influence. One part of alcohol diluted with ten thousand parts of water, is not an intoxicating drink, in any quantity which the stomach can retain: one part of alcohol diluted with one hundred parts of water, is not an intoxicating drink, unless taken in enormous quantities, or by persons highly susceptible.

The problem, in regard to the infectiousness of Cholera, is of a similar nature, and is to be solved by a reference to precisely the same three conditions, viz. dilution, quantity and susceptibility.

INFLUENCE OF DILUTION.

If several Cholera patients should at the same time occupy the same small and ill-ventilated room, the air of that room would, after some time, become so charged with the miasm, as to be capable of communicating

Cholera to other occupants, provided that by their constitution, their state of health, their neglect of regimen and of prophylactic remedies, they possessed a certain degree of susceptibility to the disease. To them, the disease would be infectious, in this concentrated state of the morbific miasm. On the other hand, if there were only one patient in a large and well-ventilated-room, the respiration of its air during the same length of time, and by individuals having the same predisposition, might be perfectly safe, and would certainly be attended with little danger as compared with that in the small, close and crowded room abovementioned. What, in a more concentrated state, was a poison, becomes comparatively innoxious by dilution. If we admit the possibility of taking Cholera under these last circumstances—if we say that even in such a room it is possible that Cholera may to some persons prove infectious, our statement is liable to be misunderstood and misapplied. One will say, Cholera is then infectious, like small-pox. This would be a gross exaggeration, and one which it is important to prevent; inasmuch as it would deter many from giving the requisite attention to the sick, and also excite, among those not yet attacked, an alarm that would increase their susceptibility. The miasm of small-pox is one that operates in a much more diluted state than that of Cholera, and requires no peculiar susceptibility except that naturally possessed by persons who have not been vaccinated. Such persons by going near a small-pox patient, even in a large and well-ventilated room, would be in great danger of taking the disease. The danger of this in case of exposure to a Cholera patient under the same circumstances, would be comparatively trifling.

Again, even the miasm of small-pox can, by diffusion in the open air, be so diluted, as to lose entirely its poisonous property, and become incapable of producing the disease. Still more easily does this take place in case of the Cholera Miasm. We have seen, that for weeks it confined itself to the hospitals at Staten-Island, without passing beyond their common enclosure to affect the village in which they are situated.

For security from infection by Cholera miasm, it must have a certain degree of dilution. Among the *practical applications* to be made of this doctrine, we may mention the importance of ventilation, of using as large rooms as possible for Cholera patients, and allowing as few patients as possible to be confined in the same room. Ventilation and washing, are the only requisites for the purification of rooms which have been occupied by Cholera patients. There is no evidence that chlorine or chloride of lime has the slightest influence on this infecting miasm itself; and the fumigation of the sick-room would be decidedly prejudicial, both to the patient and his attendants. In addition to the direct deleterious action of the gas on the system, it would interfere with the salutary action of medicines and prophylactics.

INFLUENCE OF DOSE.

Having considered the influence of dilution, I shall proceed to that of *quantity*. If any poison is diluted to that degree in which it just begins to lose its power of acting as a poison, in a certain dose, it will still act as a poison in a larger dose, or (what is nearly equivalent in practical effect) in numerous and frequently repeated doses, the aggregate of which is a very large quantity.

The Cholera miasm observes the same law. A room, occupied by Cholera patients, may be so large and well-ventilated, that a susceptible individual might be perfectly safe in it for three hours, but not for thirty. During the latter period, he would inhale ten times as much air slightly impregnated with the miasm. Allœopathic physicians have frequently seen the mischievous and even fatal effects of mercury and arsenic in what *they* call small doses, administered by them for a considerable length of time.

Still, there is nothing on earth which is a *poison*, irrespective of concentration and dose. We cannot consider the Deity as the Author of any thing which is poisonous—i. e. destructive—in its very essence. Read the impressive language of Hahnemann. "When He, the All-bountiful, created iron, He left it to the free choice of the children of men, to fashion it either into the deadly dagger, or the peaceful ploughshare, to slay or to support their race. Ah, how much happier for them, did they employ all His gifts for good! So would they fulfil His will and the end of their being. We cannot charge an all-loving Providence with the crimes, that men have committed in abusing the administration of terribly powerful drugs, by giving them in enormous doses, and in improper cases."

Such were the elevated sentiments that animated the man, who will, in all future times, be remembered as the first discoverer of a method, by which the noxious properties of the most virulent poisons may be removed, whilst their curative properties are retained or heightened. The success of this pharmaceutic method depends greatly on that minute division which is effected by a certain diluting process; yet the first object in the mind of its discoverer was the reduction of dose. He aimed to diminish the quantity of a crude allœopathic drug to such a degree, that it should cease to be a poison, that is, become a medicine fit for homœopathic use. I have been insensibly led to speak of this method, when considering the effect of inhaling a greater or less quantity of air impregnated with Cholera miasm.

Whether Cholera is or is not infectious, depends not only on the degree in which the air is impregnated with the miasm, but upon the quantity of the air inhaled, and consequently upon the length of time during which it is continuously respired.

I will make *another application* of these views, relative to the latter topic. Whereever it is practicable, there should be a provision for the occasional relief of *nurses;* so that no one should be required to spend the whole day—much less day and night—in the sick-chamber.

For making such a desirable arrangement, the homœopathic system offers peculiar advantages. In the first place, homœopathic families will have fewer cases of Cholera; secondly, these cases will be of much shorter duration, i. e. will sooner terminate in health; and thirdly, they will require less nursing in proportion to their number and duration. Every family which has enjoyed homœopathic practice, knows what an amount of nurse-labor is dispensed with by avoiding external applications, to say nothing of evacuants, which in case of Cholera the disease itself often supplies, as if to give, at the same time, a specimen and a reproof, of allœopathy carried to perfection.

INFLUENCE OF SUSCEPTIBILITY.

But not only does Cholera fail to be infectious, unless there is a sufficient concentration of the poison in the air, and a sufficient quantity of this air respired; but it also fails to be infectious, unless there is a peculiar predisposition or *susceptibility* in the person exposed. Some possess an immunity, from the very nature of their constitutions, others by the good state of their health at the time, others by the judicious regulation of their diet and regimen, and others in consequence of having taken the homœopathic prophylactics, i. e. preventive medicines.

What I have to say hereafter in regard to the success of prophylactic and therapeutic measures, is calculated to confirm the confidence and hopes of the homœopathic members of the community; and what I have said in regard to infection, is also calculated to allay anxiety. When the public are apprized, that, in the last travel of the Cholera, the first place in which it appeared on this continent, was not in any filthy street of any large city, but in a hospital into which Cholera patients had been recently introduced, it will be difficult to persuade them, that the vicinity of those already affected with Cholera, has not some influence in propagating the disease. The anxiety which such a fact is calculated to excite, is not allayed by the disputes of the faculty in regard to the question whether the disease is, or is not contagious, nor by any distinctive names, expressing merely the modes of communication. The true solace is to be derived from a consideration of the various degrees of infecting power, and the feebleness of that of Cholera; and the true security is to be derived from an examination and application of the principles, on which this infecting power is still farther enfeebled, so as to become scarcely appreciable, and from those prophylactic measures which diminish or remove individual susceptibility.

It is probable, that almost all diseases are more or less communicable to individuals who have a peculiar susceptibility to their respective influences. Some of these diseases, as small-pox, are generated by the reception of inconceivably minute doses of the morbid product. Small-pox, again, is an example of a disease which requires no special susceptibility; none which is not naturally possessed by almost all persons previously to vaccination; whereas a majority escape Cholera, even when they are most fully exposed to it, and pay no special attention to diet or regimen.

In the case of cholera, as well as of most other diseases, the liability to infection, depends vastly more upon the peculiar susceptibility of the individual, than upon the degree of exposure. When cholera is introduced into a city, a majority of its inhabitants may have symptoms which mark its presence in the atmosphere; but only a small proportion usually take the disease, however intimate their communication with the sick; and of those who do become affected with it, there is a large majority who have had no obvious and direct communication with persons laboring under the disease.

ROUTES AND MODES IN WHICH THE CHOLERA TRAVELS.

In its progress from one country to another, and from city to city, it oftener selects the great thoroughfares of men, and especially rivers. Its preference of low situations, and especially of the shores of rivers and other bodies of water, appears however not to be entirely owing to human intercourse. In 1832, I observed that nearly all the cases at the commencement of the epidemic in Schenectady, were for some time in a retired part of the town near the Mohawk, a river not used for navigation. At other times, the disease travels across dry regions, and seems to pass from city to city independently of human intercourse. Cholera, then travels by two methods; viz., with men as vehicles, and without any obvious and visible vehicles of transportation: it sometimes goes, at other times it is carried.

During its prevalence in any part of a country or of a city, some degree—more or less slight—of a widely diffused *epidemic influence*, is usually manifested, by a tendency to diseases somewhat similar, provided the season of the year is favorable to the spread of cholera.

As to quarantine regulations, we can rarely expect from them more than some postponement of the invasion. Even this will justify their rigorous enforcement. The disease is propagated partly, though not exclusively, by infection.

CHAPTER IV.

HYGIENE AND PROPHYLAXIS.

ARTICLES WHICH SHOULD NOT BE USED BY PERSONS WHO ARE TAKING HOMŒOPATHIC MEDICINES, EITHER DURING THE PREVALENCE OF THE CHOLERA OR AT OTHER TIMES.

1st. Raw vegetables—such as celery, lettuce, &c.;

2d. Unripe, or sour fruits, and acids in general;

3d. Food which has any medicinal qualities—such as onions and tomatoes, and bread prepared with soda;

4th. Coffee, green tea, and distilled and fermented liquors;

5th. Condiments (except salt), as vinegar, pickles, pepper, spices and mustard;

6th. Camphor, hartshorn, cathartics, herb-teas, and other medicines (whether external or internal) except those prescribed by the physician;

7th. Tobacco in great quantities, especially by chewing; and in any quantity unless the individual has been long accustomed to it.

None of the forbidden articles (except coffee, and camphor, and other medicines), need to be suddenly and totally abandoned, if the individual has been long accustomed to them. In that case, he may, unless forbidden by his physician, use them, though in great moderation. Great and sudden changes in regard to the use of condiments, should not be made after the epidemic has actually commenced in the place. Let the reform commence earlier.

HYGIENIC RULES IMPORTANT TO BE OBSERVED BY PERSONS IN GENERAL DURING THE PREVALENCE OF THE CHOLERA, AND USEFUL AT ALL OTHER TIMES.*

1st. Use warm clothing, and in cool or changeable weather, flannel; but put a

* The imperative form is used here for brevity.

cotton or silk garment under it, unless you have been accustomed to flannel next the skin.

2d. Avoid taking cold, or becoming chilled.

3d. Use no cold, nor hot, nor even tepid baths; but use cool baths, those which feel like a summer breeze, or sponge the body with water of such a temperature. This, with different individuals and different modes of using the water, may range from 75° to 80° Fahrenheit.

4th. Remain in the water not longer than a minute; and wash and wipe yourself dry as soon as possible; and if in the least chilly, put on extra clothing. Use this ablution once a week, or twice in summer, and wash the feet and other more sweaty parts of the body daily.

5th. Endeavor to encourage good temper, hope and cheerfulness in yourself and others.

6th. Use moderate and even active exercise, but avoid great fatigue.

7th. Avoid all kinds of fasting, when there is appetite.*

8th. Let the diet consist partly of animal food, and partly of good bread or some

* I will not deny that any man has a right to punish himself by abstaining from hurtful luxuries: but he has no right to punish himself by injuring his health.

other preparation of wheat flour.* Use a good proportion of fresh beef, mutton, venison, or fowls, and, if it agrees with the stomach, soup made of one of these meats. Fish, eggs, good milk, butter, sugar, and molasses, are not hurtful to persons in general, when used in moderation, and with a due proportion daily of some of the meats above-mentioned.

9th. Avoid all indigestible food, every thing which you have found to oppress your stomach, whether it be cabbage, turnip, or other succulent vegetables, fresh bread, rich pastry, old or toasted cheese, meat too fatty, veal or other young meats, sausages, pork, geese, lobsters, shell-fish, eels or other fish which have not both fins and scales. The articles enumerated in this paragraph are of doubtful character for most dyspeptics at all times, and for most persons when Cholera prevails.

10th. Eat with moderation: take care not to overload the stomach with food of any kind.

11. Masticate the food thoroughly. If possible, observe regular and early hours for eating and sleeping. Avoid late suppers: but if compelled to defer the evening meal till a late hour, eat sparingly.

* This last, possessing considerable azote, has some chemical similarity to animal food.

12th. Drink water, cocoa, pure unspiced chocolate, toast-water, barley-water, or weak black tea.

13th. Avoid as far as possible all alcoholic drinks, whether distilled or fermented, but especially the former. Use neither coffee nor green tea.

14th. Keep your room properly ventilated, but in such a manner as not to expose yourself to currents of air when sitting still.

15th. Do not continue long in small rooms that are crowded with people.

16th. If practicable, avoid sleeping in basements, or with many persons in the same room.

Peculiarities of constitution and inveterate habits, and the disadvantages of making great and sudden changes after the commencement of the epidemic, will justify some modification in the above rules by some individuals. In food, some concessions must be made to taste.

PROPHYLACTICS.

The homœopathic *preventives* of Cholera are *Cuprum metallicum*, and *Veratrum album*, prepared according to the homœopathic method, and taken alternately in doses of two or three pellets once or twice a week. By this means thousands have been protected from the disease. It is said, that there is no instance in which persons thus treated have fallen victims to Cholera. The globules may be placed on the tongue, and allowed to dissolve in the mouth, and then swallowed.

Wherever it is practicable, a homœopathic physician should be consulted; as one of these remedies would in some cases be preferable to the other. He could decide which.

The method which Hahnemann recommended, and which many employed with success, was to take globules medicated with the 30th dilution of *Cuprum*, then wait one week, and take the similarly medicated globules of the 30th of *Veratrum;* then after a week, the *Cuprum*, and so on. Others have used, with similar success, the third dilution of each, at intervals of half a week. This may be used by those who cannot obtain the thirtieth; but let no one venture upon the use of the copper of the drug stores, nor the crude colored tincture of veratrum, even of the homœopathic pharmacies.

The efficiency and duration of the action of a prophylactic are very great, provided it is sufficiently analogous to the disease to be prevented. We have examples in vaccination as a preventive of variola, and in belladonna as a preventive of scarlatina. Again, it is not probable that the action of attenuated medicines can be entirely frustrated by antidotes taken in the crude form. The attenuations have peculiar power. Every experienced and observant homœopathic physician knows, that less than a billionth part of a grain of common salt will manifest its specific effects in an individual who is taking many grains of crude salt at every meal. The rule of three fails to explain the effect of such an infinitessimal increase in the quantity. The inference is inevitable, that the homœopathic process has developed immense power.

Yet to those who have less confidence in the intensity and duration of the action of these attenuations, or who are not very strict in their homœopathic regimen, it might be well to take each medicine once a week, i. e. alternately at intervals of three or four days. Take the medicine in the morning on rising, an hour before breakfast; or, if at another time, take nothing in the mouth, except pure water, within an hour after taking the medicine.

When a family is to be protected, we might dissolve five or six pellets of the 12th of veratrum in a gill of clean cold water, and give each member one, two or three tea-spoonfulls, according to the age. Then after waiting three days, use the thirtieth of cuprum in the same dose and manner; then wait three days, and give the thirtieth of veratrum in the same dose and manner. Afterwards, alternate the thirtieth of each in solution as before described, and at the same intervals. I advise commencing with the veratrum, because the Cholera, and especially the present epidemic, oftener requires veratrum, at least in the male sex. Camphor is too transient in its action to be of any use as a prophylactic: besides it would interfere with other medicines. Persons who may be so circumstanced as to think it best to carry it in their pockets, to have it ready in case of attack, should keep it very tightly corked, and, unless attacked, should not use it, even by smelling, when they have been taking a prophylactic.

CHAPTER V.

HISTORY OF TREATMENT,

OR

STATISTICAL PROOFS OF THE SUCCESS OF HOMŒOPATHY IN CHOLERA.

A vast number of remedies and modes of allœopathic treatment have enjoyed ephemeral reputation, have been lauded, rejected, revived, and again rejected. This may be partly explained by the fact, that medicines and methods employed toward the close of the epidemic in any place, acquire an undue reputation, because the disease is usually at that period less malignant and fatal. The physician not appreciating this, publishes his specific in good faith; but it utterly fails with those who subsequently try it in a different place, in any stage of the epidemic in which nature is not nearly competent to the cure. There is no plan of treatment agreed upon, even by one-fourth of the allœopathic physicians, and very little confidence in allœopathic Cholera practice in general, among most of the best informed of that school. An able allœopathic author who practised in 1831 and 1832, in England, where homœopathy was then unknown, says, "If the balance could be fairly struck, and the exact truth ascertained, I question whether we should find that the average mortality from Cholera in this country, was any way disturbed by our craft. Excepting always the cases in which preliminary diarrhœa was checked, just as many, though not perhaps the very same individuals, would, probably, have survived, had no medication whatever been practised." *

A friend asks me—How will you treat the Cholera? I answer, homœopathically. I perceive he almost trembles at the thought, provided he is a new convert, and one unacquainted with the homœopathic history of this disease. I endeavor to remove his solicitude, by assuring him that there is no method of treating Cholera which can be compared with Hahnemann's. Has it ever been tried? This question is a very reasonable one. Thousands of Americans will ask

* Lectures on the Principles and Practise of Physic; delivered at King's College, London, by Thomas Watson, M. D. p. 828.

it, at a time when the Cholera is approaching them, in a form as virulent as was ever known in Europe or America, if we can judge from the loss of one half the patients, even in private practice, by the European and American allœopathists.

I will let statistics answer this question and show the relative results. Whençe the horror which the name of this disease awakens? It comes from the deplorable failure of allœopathic treatment.

The first seven cases which occurred on board the packet ship New-York, in Dec. 1848, died under calomel treatment. The ship arrived at the Quarantine at Staten-Island, near New-York, on the 2d of December, and landed the remaining eleven or twelve patients, who had survived longer under a comparatively inert treatment. From the statement of the captain, and the daily published reports of the health-officer, from Dec. 5th to Jan. 4th—when reports ceased to be published—it appears that in the ship before her arrival, and in the hospitals at the Quarantine since, there had occurred about ninety-six cases and fifty-two deaths, from Cholera.* The cases at the Quarantine were under the care of the health-officer himself, a skilful allœopathic

* I believe that the official statistics have not yet been published in any other form.

physician, who, having the population of the buildings under his supervision, had an opportunity of instructing them in regard to premonitory symptoms, and it is to be presumed, of treating them in an early stage. Yet more than one half died, under calomel and other allœopathic treatment.

There is no instance on record, of such mortality among the same number of persons under homœopathic treatment, for Cholera, or for *any acute disease whatever*, in any part of the world.

But as ratios obtained from large numbers are more reliable for showing the true average, I shall confine myself to the Cholera of 1831—1832.

In 1832 there were in this city—including Bellevue—5232 cases, of which 2031 died; i. e. nearly one out of every 2½ or 2⅔, or in round numbers, nearly 2 out of 5. Of persons treated at their homes, there were 2859 cases, of whom 937 died; i. e. about one in every 3 persons attacked. In the hospitals—including Bellevue—there were 2373 cases, and 1094 deaths; i. e. nearly one half died. Such were the best results that could be obtained here by allœopathic skill. There is a close resemblance between this result and that of the present year as above stated. The malignity of the disease and the impotence of allœopathic art, remain the same. In Europe, in 1831—1832, this disease, under allœopathic treatment, was still more fatal. In the allœopathic hospitals of Italy and France, in 21 of which I have seen the ratio of death stated, the average of the ratios gives 63 deaths out of every 100 patients.

The only treatment which proved itself worthy of any confidence, was the homœopathic. It is not denied by allœopathists themselves, that it was the great success that attended the homœopathic treatment of Cholera in Europe, that gave this system the most powerful impulse that it has ever received. Dr. Balfour of Edinburgh, who is opposed to the system, writes to Dr. Forbes from Vienna in 1836, in the following words: "During the first appearance of Cholera here, the practice of homœopathy was first introduced; and Cholera, when it came again, renewed the favorable impulse previously given, as it was through Dr. Fleischmann's successful treatment of this disease, that the restrictive laws were removed, and homœopathists obtained leave to practise and dispense medicines in Austria. Since that time their number has increased more than threefold in Vienna and its provinces." He also says: "No young physician settling in Austria—excluding government officers—can hope to make his bread, unless at least prepared to treat homœopathically, if requested."

In statistics, I shall confine myself to the epidemic of 1831—1832, it being the most severe, and the only one whose statistics are tolerably complete. Let no one trust his life to any vaunted method of cure which has been tried only on a few scores of patients, and by one or two physicians. The homœopathic method has been tried on many thousands of Cholera patients, and with a success remarkably uniform in different countries.

Let us compare the results of the two systems in the same city. In Vienna, there were 4500 patients treated allœopathically; of whom 1360 died. There were 581 treated homœopathically; of whom only 49 died. This gives 31 per cent. of deaths under the former, and only 8 per cent. under the latter.

Dr. Quin of London has given a table of the results of the treatment of ten different homœopathic physicians. The worst result under any of these physicians was, the death of only one-fifth of his patients, whilst four-fifths were saved. The best result obtained by any one of these physicians was the saving of 40 out of every 41, or losing 3 out of 125, this being the number of cases which he treated. This physician was Dr. Weith of Vienna. These cures were made at a time when this pestilence was prevailing in that city in its greatest intensity, and baffling all the skill of alloeopathic physicians.

The statements of this venerable man can be relied on. He is above suspicion. He had no party prejudices to mislead him; no professional interests to advance. Though he had taken the degree of Doctor of medicine, his profession was that of a minister of religion. But when he beheld his fellow-citizens doomed to destruction, his feelings as a man, and his principles as a christian, impelled him to stretch forth his arm for their relief. He had just become convinced of the truth of the homœopathic doctrine, and of its practical importance. It was distressing to him, to be continually called to the death-beds of persons who might have been saved by homœopathy, but were perishing in spite of allœopathy. His spirit was stirred within him, and he resolved to suspend in part and for a time his functions as the spiritual guide of his people, and devote himself to their temporal salvation. He acted as a true disciple of Him, who delighted in saving not only the souls but the lives of men.

The efforts of Dr. Weith were crowned with a success fully justifying the expectations which he had been led to entertain by the success of other homœopathic physicians in this same epidemic.

The remedies which he employed, were

Phosphoric acid, *Veratrum*, *Cuprum*, Tincture of *Camphor*, and under some circumstances, lavements of ice-water.

Of the 1093 patients, treated by the ten homœopathic physicians, 998 were saved, and only 95 lost. Thus the average proportion of deaths was only one to 11½, or 2 out of 23 patients, whilst 21 out of 23 patients were saved. The results above-stated were chiefly obtained at Vienna, in Moravia, Bohemia and Hungary, during the epidemic of 1831 and 1832. Dr. Rath, who had been sent, in April, 1832, by order of the king of Bavaria, to collect authentic information, respecting the results of the homœopathic treatment of the Cholera, reported officially the several results of the treatment of 14 homœopathic physicians at Prague, in Moravia, in Hungary and at Vienna. The total number of cases which he reported was 1269; cures, 1184, deaths, 85.

In Russia and Austria, and at Berlin and Paris, there were 3017 cases treated homœopathically; of which 2753 were cured, and only 264 died; i. e. only about one in 11½ died. On an average more than 10 out of 11 were cured.

Hon. Alexis Eustaphieve, the Russian Consul General, has given the results obtained by homœopathic treatment in various parts of the Russian Empire, in 1830 and 1831. Of 70 patients treated in two places, all were cured. The total result was, that of 1270 patients, 1162 were saved, and only 108 lost; showing an average proportion of one death in 11¾. This agrees remarkably with the success obtained in other countries.

These facts are derived from the reports of Admiral Mordvinow, then President of the Imperial Council, who affirms, that "Not a single death has occurred where Homœopathic treatment was resorted to in the incipient symptoms of the Cholera;" and that "it was remarked, that all the patients cured by Homœopathia, regained, in a very short time, their former health and strength; while those who survived other treatments, were left in a state of weakness which lasted several months, and but too often terminated in another disease which proved fatal."

The following is an extract from a letter which Admiral Mordvinow received from his daughter, Madame Lvoff, of the government of Saratow. It is dated August 6th, 1831.

"The dreadful Cholera broke out last month in our own village and its vicinity with the greatest fury. My husband was the first person attacked; but thanks to Homœopathia, was cured in a few days. From a desire to relieve the sufferings of humanity, he visited all the places in the neighborhood, wherever the disease raged the most; administered the remedies; instructed the priests and the elders in the use of them; and was whole weeks thus employed, while I remained at home occupied with the preparation of Homœopathic powders. Four hundred Cholera patients, saved and restored to perfect health, was the gratifying reward of his zeal, and the triumphant result of Homœopathic doses liberally distributed to all who applied for them. We are all now so well convinced of the miraculous power of this system, that we cannot sufficiently deplore the ignorance that *cannot*, and still more the obstinate prejudice that *will not* invoke its aid, and thereby rescue relatives and friends from certain death. The Asiatic Cholera, preceded by terror, ushered in by danger, and followed by desolation, comes now, remains, and departs a harmless thing. Its cure is in reality easier than that of a fever. Multiplied experiments, and consequent confidence in Homœopathic treatment, have divested it of all its appalling attributes, by subjugating it entirely to the skill of man. We had fifty patients in our own village, and not *one* of them *died*. On the estate of my sister-in-law, there were likewise a good many *cases*, but no *deaths*. There is also an abundance of reason to believe that the fatal termination of the disease, wherever it occurred, was occasioned altogether by neglect, want of necessary precaution, or deviation from the rules of regimen prescribed by Homœopathia. All the sick who took medicine in strict conformity to the rules, were *saved*, although some of them were already in the state of collapse, which apparently precluded all hope. In this last stage there were not a few with their teeth clenched so fast that it was necessary to force them open for the purpose of introducing the medicine; and yet, on the very day following, they were relieved and convalescent! My good husband, from the constant intercourse with the sick, took the infection several times, but in every instance was restored by a few Homœopathic globules. In short, we consider ourselves perfectly safe from this dreaded scourge, whatever may be its potency and virulence. The repeated numerous trials have more than satisfied us, that in the presence of Homœopathia, with its five remedies only, the Asiatic Cholera is not a mortal disease, and still less so when encountered at its commencement."*

* "Homœopathia Revealed," by the Hon. Alexis Eustaphieve. Mr. Eustaphieve has a copy of the original documents. I find in the "Bibliothèque Homœopathique," the same extract, with a very few slight verbal discrepancies.

There are informal accounts from Petersburgh and Riga, of relative success, in the Homœopathic treatment of the Cholera of 1848, similar to that which distinguished that treatment in former years. There have been employed with great effect, Camphor, Carbo-vegetabilis, Jatrapha curcas, Hydrocyanic acid, Phosphoric acid, Veratrum, etc. Veratrum is said to have gained great renown, even among Allœopathists themselves, when they witnessed its effects in the hands of Homœopathic physicians. But the statistics of Homœopathic practice in the Cholera of 1848 have not yet been published.

To the statistics above given, in relation to the first invasion of this disease, I need not add a word of comment, to show the immense superiority of the Homœopathic treatment. Such a uniformity in the results in so many places, and with such a number of patients, must speak convincingly to every intelligent and unprejudiced mind. Some of our Allœopathic brethren—as if conscious of the weakness of their system, on the broad field of extensive statistics, are at present restricting themselves to a guerilla warfare. When a single death occurs among the patients of the 50 homœopathic physicians of our city, it is noised abroad as something remarkable. But if any one is desirous of knowing the true relative value of the two systems, he must examine the subject on a broader scale. He must consider the number which Homœopathy cures, in this city and throughout the world, and the average relative results of the two methods of treatment.

CHAPTER VI.

EARLY TREATMENT,

INCLUDING THAT OF THE PREMONITORY SYMPTOMS, AND OF THE DISEASE AT ITS ONSET, WITH DIRECTIONS FOR THE GENERAL MANAGEMENT.

TREATMENT OF PREMONITORY SYMPTOMS.

During the prevalence of Cholera in a place, every person should consult his physician for such slight symptoms as often precede Cholera. By so doing, an attack may almost always be prevented, if the physician is a Homœopathist. The most usual premonitory symptom, is a slight diarrhœa, which would cause no apprehension in ordinary times. This is cured by *Camph.*^{3}, *Phosphorus*^{30}, *Phosphoric acid*^{30}, or *Veratrum*^{30}, given in the mode which I shall describe under the first variety of Cholera. When this diarrhœa is a little more marked, and but few other symptoms present, the case is usually named *Cholerine*. This case is intermediate between that of premonitory symptoms, and that of the fully formed Cholera of the first variety to be described. It requires similar treatment, and especially *Camph.*^{3}, followed by Phosphorus, *Phosphoric acid*, or *Veratrum*; the last if there is colic, vertigo, and yellow coat on the tongue.

For other premonitory symptoms, and for the cases in which *Veratrum* is preferable, consult the succeeding chapters, including the Repertory. Where there is diarrhœa, without any special indication for any particular remedy, give one drop of spirits of *Camphor*, on a lump of sugar or in sugared water. Give another drop after one hour,—or earlier, if the diarrhœa returns—and let it be followed by three doses of the 3d attenuation of Camphor, at intervals of an hour, or after each evacuation, if it occurs sooner; after this, if the diarrhœa continues, give *Phosphorus* or *Phosphoric acid*, or other remedies, according to the indications.

The *Camphor* may also be used for a short time, with advantage for most *other premonitory symptoms;* but if this is domestic treatment, there should be no unnecessary delay in consulting a Homœopathic physician; as the disease may reach a dangerous height before the appropriate remedy is employed.

In giving pellets of any medicine, in the dry state, a good general rule is: Put two or three pellets in a small powder of pure sugar or sugar of milk, fold the paper, then mash the pellets, then open the paper, and mix them by moving the paper without touching the powder. Then with the paper bent at an angle, place its edges in contact with the upper lip or teeth, let the powder slide on the tongue without touching it with the paper. The patient should hold his head back, his mouth open, and his tongue out, and allow the powder to dissolve on the tongue before swallowing it.

Where a number of doses of any one medicine are to be given in succession, it is more convenient and equally effectual to dissolve five or six pellets in a gill of water, and give one, two or three teaspoonfuls—according to the patient's age—at a dose. This may be considered as applying to any case, in this or any other stage.

TREATMENT AT THE COMMENCEMENT OF CHOLERA IN ALL ITS FORMS.

When there is a decided attack of Cholera, we resort for the first hour—or a longer or shorter time, according to circumstances—to a treatment for which—as well as for all the most successful modes of preventing and curing this disease—the world is indebted to Hahnemann.

Whatever may be the form of the attack, give one drop of the tincture of Camphor, dropped on a lump of sugar, and then dissolved in a tablespoonful of cold water. Repeat this every five minutes, until there is a decided mitigation of the symptoms. This will usually be after 5 or 6 doses. One sign of its good effect is perspiration. In proportion as the symptoms yield, let the doses be at longer intervals, as an hour, two hours, twelve and even 24 hours. For these later doses, the 3d attenuation would probably be preferable. If the disease is taken in time, 10 or 12 doses of the tincture are ordinarily sufficient. If the stomach will not retain the camphor, even in ice water, then give, before and after it, a bit of ice as large as a filbert.

In the preparation of this spirits of camphor, Hahnemann recommended the proportion of one oz. of solid camphor (the gum as it is called) to twelve of alcohol. Dr. Quin used the proportion of one to six. The usual tincture of the shops is suitable.

The most convenient method—and one which I have recently employed in a case of severe spasmodic Cholera—is to put twelve drops of camphorated spirits in a tablespoonful of sugar, and dissolve it in twelve tablespoonfuls of cold water in a tumbler, and give a tablespoonful of this mixture every five minutes till relief is obtained. Where there is great difficulty in retaining fluids on the stomach, let the medicine be so dissolved that a teaspoonful shall be a dose.

Families should be provided with the camphor, and in case of attack, administer it immediately, before the arrival of the physician, who will judge whether it is to be continued. In some cases of severe spasms, it might perhaps be admissible to give the camphor every 3d minute, till there was some mitigation. But the advantages of the camphor treatment cannot be secured by Allœopathic doses, whether at short or long intervals. In the former case, the disease would be aggravated; and in the latter case, the medicinal action would become exhausted: in both cases, the stomach would be irritated. If one ignorantly attempts to correct this last effect by combining opium or laudanum with the camphor, he, in a great measure, destroys the efficacy of the latter, besides doing direct and positive injury by the opiate.

There is abundant testimony to the efficacy of the pure camphor treatment (by small doses) from all parts of Europe.

Hahnemann states, that at Berlin and Magdeburg alone, thousands of families having followed his instructions respecting the treatment by camphor, restored those of their members who were attacked by the epidemic—restored them often in less than a quarter of an hour.

Dr. Quin assures us, that this method may be employed with certainty of success in the first hour; with probability in the following hours.

Hahnemann at first advised the external, in connexion with the internal, use of camphor, but subsequently found it unneces sary. Indeed it not only is useless, but fills the room with effluvia which interfere with subsequent treatment.

But as it is often difficult to persuade the friends of the patient to wait for the action of the remedy, they may be allowed to rub with a flannel, either dry, or moistened with alcohol, or—what is better—with their dry hands. They may also be allowed to place a warm brick at the feet of the patient—if they are cold—although it is of no positive use.

DIRECTIONS FOR THE GENERAL MANAGEMENT OF A CHOLERA PATIENT.

1. Apply no camphor externally, and use no external applications of any kind.

2. Give no drinks but cold water, unless the patient prefers warm toast water, which is the case in but very few instances.

3. Ice water may be taken as frequently as the patient desires it. It is useful for extreme thirst, cramps, colic, vomiting and cold skin.

4. The food should consist of mutton or chicken broth, with no seasoning except a moderate quantity of salt. Beef broth will answer. Oyster soup is not allowed. Great care should be used in regard to diet during convalescence.

5. The patient should lie in bed, with comfortable coverings.

6. If the weather is cool, there should be a good fire, which will allow the windows to be kept open for ventilation.

7. The patient should not, however, be exposed to cold air. If compelled to rise, he should be covered, and the windows closed.

8. He should rise no oftener, and move no more, than necessary; as motion is hurtful. He should, if practicable, be provided with a bed-pan, instead of being compelled to rise.

9. No glass or spoon which has been used for one medicine, should be used for another, until it has been rinsed with clean hot water, (without soap,) then, whilst hot, wiped dry with a clean towel, and allowed to stand till cool, and thus become more perfectly dried by its own heat. Or when convenient, it should be washed with hot water, and wiped, then heated near a fire, and again allowed to cool before being used for another medicine.

CHAPTER VII.

SYMPTOMS AND TREATMENT OF THE VARIETIES OF THE CHOLERA.

LAW OF CURE, AND REPETITION AND MAGNITUDE OF DOSES.

The skilful Homœopathic physician does not neglect the teachings of clinical experience; but he relies mainly on the law, that any disease, in its curable stage, can be cured by a medicine which is capable of producing a sufficiently large group of symptoms similar to those which the disease itself presents. Judgment is required in regard to the relative importance of symptoms; but it is important to consult repertories and materia medicas with regard to a great number of the symptoms of a case, and to combine as many as possible, and thus eliminate the false remedies and arrive at the true remedy for the whole group, and consequently for the disease of which that group is the index or exponent. The popular error, that a knowledge of the name, essential nature and principal seat of the disease, is prerequisite to a successful treatment of it, is founded upon the blind nature of Allœopathic therapeutics. Allœopathy has no guide but the name, the supposed nature and the supposed seat of the malady: and if any one who has received some Homœopathic light, allows himself to be still led by the blind, he will fall into the same ditch.

The usual intervals between the doses of attenuated medicines for the more severe varieties of Cholera are, half an hour, one hour, and an hour and a half, according to the violence of the disease.

In some violent cases, the medicine may be repeated in fifteen minutes. But we are not to suppose that the good effect is ordinarily increased by this greater frequency, or that too frequent a repetition is harmless. Again, we are not to suppose, that the operation of an attenuated medicine will be frustrated by the occurrence of vomiting at the end of several minutes after it has been swallowed. It is not like a crude drug. Some portion of it has already gone to every part of the body; and the portions which have entered the circulation have nearly as much power as the whole dose. In regard to dose and mode of administration, consult Chap. VI.

The proper attenuations for the respective medicines are stated in the Introduction. They are, in most of them, the 12th or 30th. They may be given dry, in loaf sugar or sugar of milk, or in solution in iced water. Iced water is itself a remedy, and it may be given to the patient in most cases. In regard to the repetition of attenuated medicines, a rule applicable to all cases of Cholera is—discontinue the administration of medicine as soon as there is amendment, and as long as this is progressive.

In the case of camphor, as compared with other medicines, the dose is large and the repetitions frequent; for it is unlike all other medicines in not requiring attenuation and in being exceedingly transient in its action. Hahnemann directed one drop of the tincture every five minutes; the tincture being made by dissolving one oz. of camphor in 12 of alcohol. Dr. Quin happened to use, in his own case, two-drop doses, of the tincture made in the proportion of one to six, and finding it to succeed, used it for others. Hartmann recommends the proportion of one to twenty, and the dose one or two drops, every two or five minutes. The tincture directed by the Allœopathic pharmacopœias and found in the drug-stores, is generally one to eight, sometimes one to sixteen. There is probably no better rule, than to dissolve 1 oz. of camphor in 10 oz. (i. e. 2½ gills) of alcohol.* The ordinary dose will be one drop every five minutes. In some cases, the dose may be increased to two drops, or the intervals reduced to two or three minutes. Give the tincture in sugared water, iced or at least cold. As camphor is one of the most powerful and general antidotes to other medicines, the patient must not take these from any glass or spoon which has contained it, nor must the odor of it be in the room after he commences other medicines.

* This is the strength of the tincture which the publisher (Wm. Radde) will sell with this book.

The forms described in this Chapter are those which the Cholera most frequently presents. Some of them are occasionally combined. The Homœopathic physician will know how to adapt his treatment to the different shades and combinations of these varieties.* He will apply the Materia Medica, and the law similia similibus curantur. The accompanying Repertories, especially that of Chapter IX., will aid in the selection of the remedies.

SYMPTOMS OF THE FIRST VARIETY, CHOLERA DIARRHŒICA—INTESTINAL OR DIARRHŒIC CHOLERA.

This is the form in which *diarrhœa* is a prominent symptom. At first there is a simple diarrhœa or one preceded by headache. There is pain in the neck and arms; lassitude in the legs; rumblings; tongue moist, a little coated, the coat oftener whitish; sometimes it is pasty, or gluey, so as to adhere to the finger when applied to it. The evacuations, at first composed of fœcal matters, shortly become yellowish, greenish or watery, sometimes red: after

* The term varieties, is not used in this book to denote unusual forms of this disease, but the more usual forms of the Cholera considered as itself a species.

a few hours or a few days, they have the appearance of barley water, rice water, or of whey with little flocks of soap distributed through it, or of milk-porridge mixed with water. The whiteness appears to depend on minute flocculi of whitish mucus, with some larger lumps of the same, sometimes as large as a pepper-corn and of a yellowish-white color. Each stool is preceded by great noise and movements in the intestines. There is a livid circle around the eyes, failure of strength, and nausea; sometimes, in a more advanced stage, vomiting and spasms.

If this form of Cholera—although it should amount only to a slight cholerine—is mistaken for an ordinary diarrhœa and improperly treated, there is great danger of its suddenly assuming a much graver form: vomiting and violent spasms may set in, and collapse and death close the scene. This alarming revolution in the disease may occur when the evacuations have not caused much debility or interfered with the usual avocations. In Europe and America, this diarrhœic form is the most frequent, especially in places and times in which Cholera does not rage in its greatest intensity. The more perfect and severe forms give no such warning, even in Europe and America.

In one sense, the premonitory diarrhœa

is a part of the diarrhœic variety of Cholera. If a line can be drawn between them, it is probably where the discharges change from the fœcal to the liquid character. The treatment is similar.

TREATMENT OF CHOLERA DIARRHŒICA.

If *Camphor* does not soon give relief, we are to resort to other medicines, generally to *Phosphorus*, *Phosphoric acid* or *Veratrum.* I have employed them all with success. The *Phosphoric acid* is to be preferred when there is a gluey matter on the tongue, or cramps in the upper arm or fore arm or in the wrists or hands, or if the stools are yellowish and the evacuations painless. Give *Phosphorus* when there is a white or a brown coat on the tongue and the evacuations attended with griping or colicky pains, or with nausea. Give *Veratrum* when the coat on the tongue is yellow and the diarrhœa painful. In some cases, *Chamomilla*, *Mercurius*, or *Secale* may be indicated.

However, Phosphorus, Phosphoric acid or Verat., generally cure; and they may often be given at first, without the previous administration of camphor, in this form of Cholera. When the evacuations are very copious, liquid and frequent, camphor should not be given many times, if at all. Put two or three globules of the 30th attenuation of *Phosphorus*, or of the 3d attenuation of *Phosphoric acid*, in a little sugar of milk, and place them on the patient's tongue; or give them in solution, in the manner described in Chapter VI. After two or three doses of phos.-ac. 3, if the indications for phos.-ac. remain, it will often be useful to employ the 30th. One dose of the 3d is, however, usually sufficient to effect a cure. Dr. Quin rarely found it necessary to give a second dose, and never till the following day. A dose of the appropriate remedy might be given after each evacuation, if it is copious, or every second evacuation, if they are small.

SYMPTOMS OF THE SECOND VARIETY, CHOLERA GASTRICA—GASTRIC CHOLERA.

This form of Cholera is characterized by frequent or almost continual *vomiting*, but is often accompanied by many symptoms of other varieties. The matters at first thrown out consist of the food which the stomach happened to contain, or the liquids which had been swallowed. They are usually thrown up with a sudden jerk without previous retching. The vomiting is sometimes preceded for a short time by nausea. There is no diarrhœa, or only one or two evacuations at the onset. The urine is scanty. The gastric variety of Cholera is neither the most frequent nor the most dangerous. When the epidemic prevails, this form may be excited by flatulent vegetables or other indigestible food.

TREATMENT OF CHOLERA GASTRICA.

The principal remedies are *Camphor*, *Ipecac.* and *Veratrum*. *Camphor* will ordinarily be proper at the onset; one drop every five minutes. If relief is not soon obtained, give *Veratrum* [12] or *Ipecac.* [3], according as one or the other is more indicated, (by the character, conditions, or concomitants of the vomiting,*) and at the usual intervals. If, by the effect of the veratrum or ipecac., the vomiting cease, but the other symptoms remain, and there is great weight at the stomach and pains in the intestines and head, then have recourse to *Nux* [30]. But if the disease is not checked, give *Verat.* [30], or other medicines according to the indications. To Cholera

* Vide the Cholera Repertory, to decide between these, or to determine whether some other remedy is preferable.

excited by anger, and attended with either vomiting or diarrhœa, *Cham.* [12] is appropriate.

SYMPTOMS OF THE THIRD VARIETY, CHOLERA SPASMODICA—SPASMODIC CHOLERA.

This form is especially characterized by *cramps* and other *spasms.* The principal symptoms are, contractions and cramps in the toes and fingers; afterwards, cramps in the calves, or convulsive movements in the muscles of the fore arm, and legs; then spasms in the upper arms and thighs, and sometimes fixed spasms in the chest, neck, and jaw, resembling those of locked jaw or tetanus. The constriction of the chest is preceded by vomiting. Neither vomiting nor diarrhœa frequently occur in this variety; but it may succeed a neglected diarrhœa, and be ushered in by a single copious vomiting, and attended by occasional retchings.

In some cases, there are first cramps in the calves of the legs; then tonic spasms of the whole of both inferior extremities, soon extending in succession to the abdomen, stomach, chest and throat; the inferior limbs remaining spasmodically extended and extremely stiff and hard, and affected with excruciating pain; a hard swelling at the stomach; spasms of the muscles of the jaw, attended with grating of the teeth; respiration almost arrested; sense of extreme suffocation; apprehension of impending dissolution; deglutition difficult, sometimes impossible. The spasms at length relax, and the patient, for a few minutes, is free from pain. Then the spasms and the pain return with their former severity.

TREATMENT OF CHOLERA SPASMODICA.

The principal remedies are *Camphor*, *Cuprum* and *Veratrum*. Give a drop of *Camphor* every five minutes. During the paroxysms, if they are extremely severe, we may give two drops at a dose, or repeat one drop every two or three minutes. The remedy next to be employed for removing the remains of the spasms and preventing their return is ordinarily Cuprum [30]. Give it in solution, or dry in doses of two or three globules, and repeat it many times at *intervals* of half an hour, or an hour, if its salutary effect is not manifested. If necessary, then give *Veratrum* (12th then 30th) in repeated doses, or other medicines according to the different indications. Cuprum may be given at the onset of the spasms, provided their character and concomitants indicate its use decidedly more than that of camphor. Vide Cholera Repertory.

SYMPTOMS OF THE FOURTH VARIETY, CHOLERA SICCA, DRY CHOLERA.

There is *no diarrhœa nor vomiting*. There is a *sudden prostration* of the vital powers; the urine is suppressed; tongue sometimes blue or blackish; the eyes up-turned and fixed; coldness of the surface of the whole body, which becomes covered with a cold, sticky sweat; the face and limbs have a violet blue color. The voice and pulse fail. This variety requires the most prompt attention.

TREATMENT OF CHOLERA SICCA.

The first remedy—as in other varieties of Cholera—is *Camphor*. In this variety, it is especially required, for arousing the nervous system. Repeat it in doses of one or two drops, every five minutes. Then, if necessary, give Veratrum every half hour, or hour, or hour and a half. If the cramps and vomitings have entirely ceased, if the patient is cold, blue and pulseless—i. e. collapsed—*Carbo v.* ^{30}, two or three globules. In this state of complete asphyxia, some recommend hydrocianic acid, 3d attenuation, every hour or two. We recognise the effect of these medicines by the pulsations becoming sensible, and sometimes by a return of the cramps, vomitings or diarrhœa; symptoms which are then to be treated by *Veratrum* or *Cuprum*, or some other remedy, according to the indication.

SYMPTOMS OF THE FIFTH VARIETY, CHOLERA ACUTA, ACUTE CHOLERA.

This variety we might call *cerebral*, as the brain, in the first stage, seems to be oppressed. Yet in its course it simulates the form of some other varieties, and like them, unless checked, ends in asphyxia and death.

The patient at first feels as if he were stunned, or has a sensation of weight in the head, or vertigo; oppression of the chest; numbness of the arms and legs. Afterwards there are rumblings in the intestines; heat of the body, pulse rapid and feeble; nausea, retching or vomiting; bilious or watery diarrhœa; suppression of urine; tongue cold; voice altered; face yellowish, with a dark blue circle around the eyes; prostration; spasms, at first, in the feet and hands, afterwards extending to the arms and legs, which become dark-blue and cold; the eyes tarnished and sunk in their orbits. The diarrhœa and cramps cease, and the disease in its later stage runs into the form of dry Cholera, characterized by cold sweats, insensible pulse, and general blueness—i. e. by collapse.

TREATMENT OF CHOLERA ACUTA.

Give *Veratrum;* at first the 12th, in persons of vigorous constitution, and after three doses, the 30th, in the quantity and at the intervals before described. In cases of persons of feeble constitution, give one dose of the 12th, and follow it by as many of the 30th as shall be necessary.

If in this or any other variety of Cholera, there is severe burning in any part of the alimentary-canal, with violent colic, and great weakness or restleness, give *Arsenicum.*[30] If the colic proves obstinate, give an enema of ice-water. Though veratrum is in general the grand remedy for this somewhat complicated variety, yet it will often be necessary to consult a repertory or materia medica, and determine the remedy by groups of symptoms.

SYMPTOMS OF THE SIXTH VARIETY, CHOLERA GASTRO-ENTERICA—GASTRO-ENTERIC CHOLERA.

This is a kind of combination of the gastric and diarrhœic varieties; yet being not unfrequent in its occurrence, it merits a distinct consideration. It is characterized by vomiting and diarrhœa, almost simultaneous in their commencement and nearly equal in their intensity and duration. These evacuations from the stomach and intestines agree in another respect: viz. in consisting at first of the usual contents of those cavities respectively, (i. e. food being vomited, and fœcal matter dejected,) and in soon becoming thinner, afterwards watery, and ultimately assuming the rice-water appearance. Although this combination of upward and downward discharges is characteristic of this variety, there may be some cramps, and great coldness of the body, and the patient may be, within a few hours after the attack, in the blue and pulseless condition of collapse.

TREATMENT OF CHOLERA GASTRO-ENTERICA.

The principal remedy is *Veratrum*, in the doses and at the intervals before mentioned.

If a dose or two of the 12th is given at first, the 30th should be given subsequently.

If the treatment is commenced very early, *Camphor* will be appropriate, and ordinarily sufficient. Dose, one drop every five minutes. When the stools become exceedingly copious and liquid, veratrum is in most cases to be used. If there is a complication of other symptoms, the groups may indicate some other remedy.

SYMPTOMS OF THE SEVENTH VARIETY, CHOLERA INFLAMMATORIA—INFLAMMATORY CHOLERA.

In some small proportion of instances, Cholera is, from the commencement, an inflammatory disease. The physician will recognise this character, more especially by the state of the pulse, so different from that of Cholera in every other form. In addition to the fulness and frequency of pulse, there is great heat of the body; redness of the eyes; head-ache, vertigo, &c.; tongue dry and warm; vomiting and spasms, but less diarrhœa. The patient may die of congestion in some organ, before he enters the 3d stage.

TREATMENT OF CHOLERA INFLAMMATORIA.

We can here make but a sparing and cautious use of Camphor, but must use Veratrum, Cuprum, or Ipecac. As soon as the vomiting is controlled, Aconite is to be used, and repeated two or three times to reduce the fever. Afterwards, the organ in which the congestion or inflammation is seated, requires special attention, and the use of Bell., Bry., Canth. or Rhus., or other medicines, according to circumstances. The indications, as in all other complicated cases of Cholera, can be properly understood only by a homœopathic physician.

The foregoing varieties are in some cases well marked, in others not. There is an advantage in attending to them; though the homœopathic physician who prescribes for the symptoms, will not deem it necessary to designate the variety. This will often be impracticable, especially if he is called when the cases are so advanced as to confound varieties which were originally distinct. In one sense, the variety may change with the stage.

CHAPTER VIII.

SYMPTOMS AND TREATMENT

OF THE

STAGES OF THE CHOLERA.

A case of either of the foregoing varieties is not usually divisible into distinct, well-defined stages; but we may enumerate four stages; some of them being oftener present or more distinct or durable in one variety, and some in another. They are: 1st. *The incipient Stage*, or *Stage of Invasion:* 2d. *The Active Stage*, or *Stage of Full Development;* 3d. *The Stage of Collapse;* and 4th. *The Stage of Reaction.*

FIRST STAGE, STAGE OF INVASION.

This is usually longest in the diarrhœic variety; in which it may continue from one hour to several days. The stools, though they may be watery and whitish, are not profuse. In the gastric variety, this stage may present a transient nausea, or a few loose fœcal stools; in the spasmodic variety, diarrhœa, or one or two vomitings; in the acute variety, vertigo; in the gastro-enteric variety, nausea.

The principal *remedies* in the first stage are: *Camphor, Phosphorus, Phosphoric acid,* and *Veratrum.*

SECOND STAGE, STAGE OF FULL DEVELOPMENT.

This, in the diarrhœic variety, is characterized by the profuse or frequent rice-water evacuations; in the gastric variety, by the vomiting of similar matter; in the spasmodic variety, by severe cramps or other spasms; in the dry variety, the first two stages may be scarcely perceptible; in the acute variety, there may be a livid appearance under the eyes, vomiting, or rumblings and liquid stools. In the gastro-enteric variety, there is profuse vomiting and diarrhœa; in the inflammatory variety, a febrile pulse and acute inflammation of some important organ.

The 2d stage has one of two terminations; viz. either collapse, or convalescence.

In the 2d stage, the principal remedies are: *Arsenicum, Camphor, Cuprum, Ipecac., Jatropha, Phosphorus, Phosphoric acid,* and *Veratrum.*

THIRD STAGE, STAGE OF COLLAPSE.

This stage of collapse may have the same character in every variety of Cholera, and in its principal features it is similar in all varieties. The term collapse is used to designate a certain collection of symptoms, including pulselessness; cold, blue and shrivelled skin; the voice reduced to a whisper; the urine and other secretions suppressed, and the face presenting a certain appearance called Choleric. The term facies cholerica is used to denote a face cold, livid and shrunk, and often anxious, the eyes sunk in the orbits, and upturned, or fixed, as if in vacant staring. The vox colerica, which belongs chiefly to this stage, is a voice hoarse, feeble, whispering, or almost imperceptible.

The duration of the 3d stage, varies from two hours to two days. It has one of three terminations; viz. either death, convalescence, or a disease which is inflammatory, congestive, or typhus. When death occurs from Cholera, it is usually at the termination of the third stage, sometimes of the fourth. The return of a perceptible pulse and of warmth, although attended with a renewal of the vomiting and diarrhœa, are favorable signs; though even after this partial reaction, there may be a relapse into asphyxia.

In the third stage, the principal *remedies* are: Arsenicum, Camphor, *Carbo vegetabilis*, Cicuta, Cuprum, Hydrocianic acid, Laurocerasus, Phosphorus, Phosphoric acid, *Secale*, and *Veratrum*.

FOURTH STAGE, STAGE OF REACTION AND SECONDARY AFFECTIONS.

The secondary affections which ensue on reaction, are congestive, *inflammatory*, or *febrile*. The 4th stage proper—i. e. reaction attended with these serious diseases—has seldom any existence after a good homœopathic treatment of Cholera proper; though there will, in some cases, be dysuria. The affections to be most apprehended after allœopathic treatment, are, inflammation, or congestion of the brain, stomach, intestines, or lungs; or typhoid fever.

So far as there is a partial reproduction of the symptoms of the second stage—which had disappeared during the collapse—a recurrence to the remedies of the second stage will be necessary in the fourth.

But for the new symptoms following reaction, use other remedies. For the irritation of the bladder, attended with painful urination, use *Cantharis* 30, every hour or two, whilst the symptoms remain urgent.

In most of these *inflammations*, however, we may give two or three doses of Acon. 24, at intervals of an hour, and then follow it by the remedy adapted to the symptoms, and the organ affected; repeating this last medicine much less frequently. If it is the *brain* that is affected, the remedy will generally be *Belladonna* 30; if the *lungs*, *Bryonia* 30, in some cases followed by *Rhus* 30; if the *stomach* or *intestines*, *Nux* 30, and sometimes *Bry.* 30; if the *bladder*, *Cantharis* 30. This last is also the remedy where there is inflammation in the lower intestines, attended with burning, tenesmus, and bloody stools. For the typhus or typhoid *fever*, *Bryonia*, and sometimes *Phosphoric acid*, may be used: but the principal remedy is *Rhus radicans*.*

* I deem it due to the profession as well as to myself, to state, that the Note on this plant, inserted without my consent or knowledge, in the Appendix to the American edition of Jahr's Symptomen-Codex, is grossly incorrect, especially where it attempts to correct my botanical description of this plant in general, and of the particular plant from which I obtained the specimen for trial. This last part of the criticism is not only incorrect, but absurd; inasmuch as the botanical character of those particular leaves could be known only to myself and my respectable

I will take this occasion to make a remark on a topic, not discussed in either of the notes above referred to. The rhus tox. which Hahnemann tried, was an exotic, and hence probably did not possess as much power as a plant of the same species found growing in its native soil in America. Dr. Wallace, a scientific oculist of this city, informs me that this is the case with stramonium; and that, on the other hand, the belladonna of Europe is more powerful, in dilating the pupil, than the exotic belladonna of America. Again, if the shrub rhus tox. is a stunted variety of the same species as the vine rhus rad., there is an additional reason for doubting whether it has as much activity: furthermore, the provings afford evidence that it has not. So far as the clinical experience of many physicians for some years can show, the rhus rad. is as efficacious as rhus tox. or more so, in those cases to which the latter is applicable. Like several other physicians, I prefer it. Wherever in the repertory, the generic term *rhus* is used alone, it may be considered as including both *rhus rad.* and *rhus tox.*

medical colleagues who engaged with me in the provings, and to whom the leaves where shown. I here reaffirm the correctness of my description, as given in the Note in the Body of the same Symptomen-Codex, pages 671 and 672.

If great debility follows the Cholera, and there are no other symptoms which require special attention, the appropriate remedy is *Cinchona.* [12] The final remedy for the more complete restoration of health, will frequently be Sulph., [30] given in a single dose, and allowed to act a long time without repetition.

When a homœopathic physician is called in any stage, to any case of Cholera which *has been under allœopathic treatment*, he is first to antidote the former treatment by *Camphor*. Give it but a short time, if there is any inflammation. He can judge if other antidotes are necessary; as they frequently will be in the course of the treatment; for calomel and other crude drugs—and even the undiluted colored tinctures of the homœopathic shops—are so durable in their mischievous action, as to require for their correction, something more durable in its curative action, than Camphor.

Since the preceding chapters were put in type, I have treated a *case* by the method there described. It commenced (without previous diarrhœa) with cramp in one shoulder. Then there was vomiting of a watery liquid with mucus, part of it milky white; vertigo and deafness; painful tonic spasms in the inferior limbs, with a few liquid stools;

spasms excited by movement; lower limbs inflexible; spasms of the abdomen and stomach; only one more vomiting; the liquid spirted about two yards; spasms continued, with marbly coldness of the feet, chin, nose and tongue; face bluish-pale. *Treatment*—Camphor, one drop every five minutes, till the spasms were a little mitigated; then Cuprum ^{30}, three globules, dry, every hour. One dose cured the deafness; and two, the spasms. I had given eight doses of Camphor. The family had given five larger doses, at longer intervals, without apparent effect. This attack was in the evening of Feb. 27, 1849. I left the patient comfortable, the same evening. Next morning warmth had returned; patient sitting up; appetite fair. For two small liquid stools, I gave Verat. ^{30}, in solution, in the same dose that I have in this book advised. Next day, no return of any symptoms. Patient convalescent—I may say cured.

In the evening of Jan. 29, 1849, I treated a *case*, like the severest spasmodic Cholera described in Chap. VII. Treatment, the same as the last, with the addition of one dose of Verat. ^{12} Success, the same. Each case was reported to the resident physician, on the day after the attack.

Since the 1st edition was published, many cholera patients have been treated homœopathically in this city, and nearly all of them cured; indeed every one, so far as I have heard, who had not taken laudanum after the attack.

CHAPTER IX.

CHOLERA REPERTORY.

CONTAINING THE IMPORTANT SYMPTOMS, AND THE USUAL GROUPS, AND THE MEDICINES TYPOGRAPHICALLY DISTINGUISHED AS TO THEIR RELATIVE VALUE IN THE CHOLERA.

EXPLANATION OF THE USE OF THE REPERTORY.

Believing that the success of Homœopathic treatment in Cholera, is such, that this book will be used by many physicians who have had but little, if any, experience in this kind of practice, I deem it proper to explain the best mode of using the Repertory.

Select two important symptoms, of the case to be treated, and ascertain what remedies are common to both. If these are too numerous to be retained in the memory, write them down. Then compare this reduced list with the remedies as given in the Repertory for some other important symptom, and thus discover what remedies are common to the three. Then select a fourth, &c., and continue this process until there is only one remedy left. This will generally be the remedy for the case, especially if the symptoms selected are really the most important.

In using this method and this Repertory in the treatment of the Cholera, it will generally save labor to omit, at every step of the process, all those medicines which are not emphasized in at least one of the two lists. Such medicines will almost always be eliminated before the above process is completed. No medicine, which is printed either in small Roman letters or

Italics, in *every* place in which it occurs in this Repertory, is, in the present state of our knowledge, known to have much power in the first three stages of non-inflammatory Cholera; and hence the use of such medicines, in Cholera, except by a very skilful practitioner, would be unsafe. If such should not all be removed by the process above described, the only safe course (at least for the beginner) would be, to commence anew and repeat the above process with other important symptoms, combining them with each other and with some of those previously selected; and in general, the making of various combinations and in various orders, will give greater security in the selection of the remedy. If there are two remedies which apply to all the known symptoms of the case, the selection may be determined by the type in which their names are here printed. If the remedy is doubtful, and there is time for study, consult Jahr's Manual, especially the New.

One object in the construction of this Repertory has been to save part of the above labor, by occasionally combining the symptoms into such groups (of two or three) as the disease more frequently presents. For obtaining the remedies for these groups, the Materia Medica of Hahnemann, the Symptomen Codex and various Repertories have been consulted. The degree of emphasis has been determined by the clinical experience of the school in Cholera. I have, however, italicised some medicines which rank high for the symptom in general, but are not known to be useful in Cholera. The emphasis given to the medicines in this Repertory, has no reference to the 4th stage, nor to the inflammatory variety, except where it is so stated.

Medicines seldom used in any disease are omitted; also some for vomiting and diarrhœa, seldom used in Cholera, and found in Chapter X.

The concomitant symptoms in any one section of this Repertory, are generally arranged in the same order as the sections themselves.

MENTAL SYMPTOMS.

Anguish, anxiety or inquietude: Acon., Ars., bell., bry., Camph., Carb. v., caus., cham., *cic.*, coff., Cupr., dig., hyos., ign., ipec., kal., Lach., Laur., lyc., merc., natr., natr. m., nitr. ac., *nux*, petr., Phos., *phos. ac.*, puls., rhus, Sec., sep., *stram.*, sulph., tart., Verat.

Apathy, or indifference: *Ars.*, bell., calc., cham., chin., *cic.*, hyos., Lach., lyc., *merc.*, *natr. m.*, *phos.*, Phos. ac., sep., staph., *verat.*

Fear of Death, with internal Burnings, and tossing in the bed: ARS.

Taciturnity, or repugnance to conversation: Ars., bell., bry., calc., *cham.*, cic., coloc., cupr., ign., lach., merc., natr. m., nux, *phos. ac.*, puls., rheum, stann., staph., sulph., sulph. ac., VERAT.

HEAD.

Confusion in the head: *Acon.*, *ars.*, *bell.*, *bry.*, calc., Camph., caus., chin., dig., merc., nux, op., *phos. ac.*, puls., rheum, rhus, *sec.*, sep., sulph. ac., tart., Verat.

Heaviness, or pressure in the head: Acon., arn., *ars.*, bell., bry., calc., CAMPH., *carb. v.*, cham., chin., *cic.*, dulc., ign., *ipec.*, *lach.*, *laur.*, lyc., merc., *natr. m.*, nux op., petr, Phos., Phos. ac., puls., rheum, rhus, sep., sil., stann., sulph., *tart.*, Verat.

Vertigo: *Acon.*, ant., arn., *ars.*, *bell.*, bry., calc., CAMPH., *carb. v.*, caus., *cic.*, *cupr.*, dig., fer., graph., hep., hyos., ign., *ipec.*, *kal.*, *lach.*, *laur*, lyc., *merc.*, natr., *natr. m*, nux op., *petr.*, Phos., Phos. ac., puls., rhus, Sec., sep., sil., stram., sulph., sulph. ac., tart., thuj., VERAT.

Vertigo with *stupor*: Ars., *bell.*, bry., calc., caus.. *kal.*, Laur., lyc., merc., *natr. m.*, nux, *op.*, Phos., *phos. ac.*, puls., rhus, Sec., sil., spig., *stram.*, sulph., *tart.*, Verat.

EYES.

Eyes *sunk* in the orbits; with Livid semicircles

under them: ARS., calc., *camph.*, *cic.*, CUPR., kal., *laur.*, PHOS., PHOS. AC., SEC., sulph., VERAT.

Eyes *sunk* in the orbits; with *hoarse* voice: ARS., calc., *camph.*, *cic.*, CUPR., kal., *laur.*, PHOS., *phos. ac.*, SEC., sulph., VERAT.

Eyes *Up-turned* and *Fixed*: CAMPH., *cic.*, VERAT.

Pupils contracted: ARS., bell., *cham.*, CAMPH., *cicut.*, *nux*, *puls.*, SECAL., sep., VERAT.

FACE.

Bluish color of the face: Acon., ARS., bell., bry., CAMPH., cham., *cic.*, con., CUPR., dig., dros., hep., *hyos.*, ign., *ipec.*, lach., lyc., merc., *op.*, *phos.*, puls., samb., spong., staph., stram., tart., VERAT.

Face *bluish* and Pale: ARS., bell., bry., CAMPH., *cic.*, con., CUPR., dig., dros., hep., hyos., ign., *ipec.*, lach., lyc., merc., op., PHOS., puls., samb., spong., *stram.*, TART., VERAT.

Bluish color about the Eyes: ARS., calc., cham., *chin.*, CUPR., fer., graph., hep., ign., IPEC., kal., lach., lyc., merc., natr., nux, *oleand.*, *phos.*, PHOS. AC., *rhus*, sabin., SEC., sep., spig., staph., stram., sulph., VERAT.

Blueness under Eyes; Sleeps with eyes Open: Ipec., PHOS. AC., *sulph.*, VERAT.

Blueness of the face and lips; Coldness of the Lips: ARS., *cupr.*, VERAT.

Facies *cholerica*: ARS., *camph.*, *carb. v.*, CUPR., ipec., *laur.*, *phos.*, phos. ac., rhus, SEC., VERAT.

Face *choleric*; Voice Hoarse: ARS., *camph.*, CARB. V., CUPR., *laur.*, PHOS., *phos. ac.*, rhus, *sec.*, VERAT.

Cold Perspiration on the face: *Carb. v.*, rheum., nux, rhus, *verat.*

Cold Perspiration on the Forehead during the Evacuation: VERAT.

Cold Perspiration on the Face and Limbs: CARB. V.

Spasm of the Jaw: Bell., *cham.*, CAMPH., *cicut.*, CUPR., *hydrocy.*, lach., *laur.*, op., rhus., SEC., VERAT.

TONGUE.

Coats on the Tongue. Brown coat: Bell., CARB. v., hyos., PHOS., rhus rad., sabin., sulph.

Coat of Mucus: Bell., *cupr.*, dulc., lach., merc., PHOS. AC., puls., sulph.

Viscid coat: PHOS. AC.

White coat: Ant., arn., bell., bry., calc., *carb. v.*, *cupr.*, dig., ign., *ipec.*, *merc.*, nitr., nux, petr., puls., sabin., *sec.*, sep., sulph.

Yellowish coat: Bell., bry., *carb. v.*, cham., chin., coloc., IPEC., *nux*, plumb., puls., *rhus rad.*, *verat.*

Coldness of the tongue: *Ars.*, bell., *camph.*, *laur.*, natr. m., *sec.*, VERAT.

Coldness of the tongue and breath: *Ars.*, CARB., v., *camph.*, VERAT.

Coldness of the tongue, with *dryness* of it and of the mouth: ARS., bell., *camph.*, LAUR., SEC., VERAT.

Coldness of the tongue, with *cold sweat* on the body: *Ars.*, *camph.*, *sec.*, VERAT.

Redness of the tongue: *Ars.*, bell., bry., cham., hyos., lach., nux, rhus, stann., sulph., *verat.*

Redness of the tip of the tongue, in the inflammatory variety, or in the 4th stage: RHUS RAD.

Tongue *Red*, and coated yellow: Bry., cham., *nux*, r. rad., VERAT.

Tongue *Red;* Pulse Slow: Bell., r. rad., VERAT.

NAUSEA AND THIRST.

Nausea with *thirst:* Bell., PHOS., VERAT.

Nausea with *vertigo:* CAMPH., merc., *verat.*

Nausea with continued *pain* at the *pit* of the *stomach:* Acon., *Ars.*, bell., CAMPH., *cham.*, CUPR., merc., *natr. m.*, *nux.*, PHOS., puls., rhus., *sulph.*, *tart.*, VERAT.

Nausea with *diarrhœa:* Ars., ipec., *merc*, PHOS.

Thirst, violent: Acon., ARS., bry., CAMPH., CARB. v., cham., *cic.*, CUPR., *ipec*, *laur.*, *merc.*, *natr. m.*, nux., *phos.*, *phos. ac.*, SEC., *stram.*, VERAT.

Thirst, with *nausea:* PHOS., VERAT.

11*

VOMITING.

Vomiting Frothy: VERAT.

Vomiting of a *watery* liquid analogous to that of the stools with pieces of *mucus:* ARS., bell., camph., CUPR., JATROPH., *sec.* IPEC., stram., VERAT.

Vomiting after *drinking:* Arn., *ars.*, bry., *nux*, puls., VERAT.

Vomiting with *pain* in the *stomach:* *Ars.*, bry., *camph.*, CUPR., IPEC., *lach.* nux., PHOS., sulph., stram., TART., VERAT.

Vomiting with *Colic:* *Ars.* CUPR., *nux*, PHOS., puls., stram., tart., VERAT.

Vomiting, with *diarrhœa:* *Ars.*, *cupr.*, *jat.*, IPEC., *phos.*, stram., tart., VERAT.

Vomiting with *Colic* and *Diarrhœa:* ARS., CUPR., PHOS., stram., tart., VERAT.

Vomiting with *lassitude:* *Ars.*, *camph.*, IPEC., phos., VERAT.

PAINFUL SENSATIONS AT THE STOMACH AND PIT OF THE STOMACH.

Burning in the stomach: ARS., bell., bry., camph., canth., CARB. v., cham., cic., jat., LAUR., merc., nux, PHOS., *phos. ac.*, SEC., *verat.*

Burning in the pit of the stomach: Acon., ARS., bell. bry., *laur.*, merc., nux., PHOS., *sec.*, VERAT.

Burning Heat in the stomach or pit of stomach: ARS., CAMPH., HYDROC., PHOS.

Burning sensation in the stomach and intestines, sometimes extending along the œsophagus to the mouth: ARS.

Cramp in the stomach: Bell., bry., *carb. v.*, cham., CUPR., natr. m., nux, PHOS., SEC., VERAT.

Pressure and Anxiety at the pit of the stomach: ARS., CAMPH., *cupr.*, IPEC., NUX VOM., *verat.*

Continued *Pain* at the Pit of the stomach with *nausea:* *Acon.*, *ars.*, *bell.*, CAMPH., *cham.*, CUPR., merc., *natr. m.*, *nux*, PHOS, rhus, *sulph.*, *tart.*, VERAT.

Pain in the stomach, *with vomiting:* *Ars.*, camph., CUPR., IPEC., PHOS., TART., VERAT.

Continued *Pain* in the *pit* of the *Stomach with Rumblings* in the intestines: Acon., bell., *camph.*, KARB. V., CUPR.,

JATROPH., merc., natr. m., *nux*, PHOS., PHOS. AC., *rhus*, SEC., *sulph.*, *tart.*, VERAT.

Aching or *pressive pain* at the *pit* of the *stomach*, *with liquid stools*: *Ars.*, CAMPH., *cupr.*, PHOS., *sec.*, *tart.*, VERAT.

Aching or *pressive pain* at the *pit* of the *stomach*, *with cramps* or other *spasms* in the *extremities* or elsewhere: CAMPH., CUPR., *phos.*, *phos. ac.*, natr. m., *sec.*, *tart.*, VERAT.

Painful *Sensibility* of the *pit* of the *stomach*, with *spasms* of the extremities: *Ars.*, CAMPH., CUPR., natr. m., *phos.*, *phos. ac.*, tart., VERAT.

ABDOMEN.

Rumblings in the intestines: Acon., *ars.*, bell., *bry.*, *canth.*, CARB. V., *cupr.* JATROPH., laur., *lyc.*, merc., *natr. m.*, *nux*, PHOS PHOS. AC., *plumb.*, *puls.*, rhus, *sec.*, stram., sulph., tart., VERAT.

Rumblings in the intestines, with continued *pain* in the *pit* of the *Stomach*: Acon, bell., *camph.*, CARB. V., CUPR., JATROPH., merc., natr. m., *nux*, PHOS., PHOS. AC., *puls.*, *rhus*, SEC., sulph., *tart.*, VERAT.

Rumblings in the intestines, *with liquid stools*: *Ars.*, JATROPH., nux, *petr.*, PHOS., PHOS. AC., puls., rhus, *sec.*, sulph., tart., VERAT.

Pains in the *abdomen*, *with diarrhœa*: ARS., *cham.*, IPEC., *laur.*, *merc.*, *merc. c.*, natr. m., nux, *phos.*, rhus, stram., sulph., tart., VERAT.

DIARRHŒA.

Diarrhœa, with a *pasty tongue*, which *sticks* to the fingers: PHOS. AC.

Diarrhœa with *nausea*: ARS., ipec., *merc.*, PHOS.

Diarrhœa with *vomitings*: *Ars.*, *cupr.*, JAT., IPEC., PHOS., stram., tart., VERAT.

Diarrhœa, with *vomiting* of the Food eaten, and of Watery liquid: ARS., CUPR., IPEC., PHOS., VERAT.

Diarrhœa, with aching or *pressure*, at or near the *pit* of the *stomach*: CAMPH., cham., CUPR., merc., natr. m., PHOS., PHOS. AC., *sec.*, VERAT.

Diarrhœa, *with pain in the abdomen*: ARS., *cham.*, IPEC. *laur.*, *merc.*, *merc. c.*, natr. m., *phos.* stram., sulph., tart., VERAT.

Stools brown: Ars., CAMPH., merc. c., sulph., *tart.*, VERAT.

Stools *greenish: Ars.*, bell., canth., *cham.*, ipec., *laur.*, *merc.*, nux, PHOS., PHOS. AC., sulph., VERAT.

Stools *grey*, or slightly whitish: Acon., *ars.*, bell., carb. v., cham., lach., merc., PHOS., PHOS. AC., puls., rhus, sulph., *verat.*

Stools *liquid:* Arn., *ars.*, *carb. v.*, chin., *cic.*, JAT., lach., *meph.*, PHOS., PHOS. AC., SEC., VERAT.

Stools *liquid* and *whitish: Ars.*, *camph.*, cupr., *jatroph.*, PHOS., PHOS. AC., *sec.*, VERAT.

Liquid and *whitish* stools, with *white* coat of *tongue: Cupr.*, PHOS., SEC.

Liquid stools, with continued *pain* at the *pit* of the *stomach: Ars.*, CAMPH., chin., *cupr.*, PHOS., VERAT.

Liquid stools, with *rumblings in the intestines: Ars.*, JATROPH., nux, petr., PHOS., PHOS. AC., puls., rhus, *sec.*, sulph, tart., VERAT.

Stools *liquid;* evacuation *painful* (attended with colic): ARS., *carb. v.*, PHOS., spig., staph., VERAT.

Stools liquid; evacuation *painless:* ARS., carb. v., chin., *cic.*, PHOS., PHOS. AC., SEC., spig., VERAT.

Stools *mucous* and *watery:* Ars., bell., chin., *ipec.*, nux, PHOS., PHOS. AC., puls., rhus SEC., sulph. ac., *tart.*, VERAT.

Rice-water stools, or stools like *whey* or water, with *Whitish* or greyish *flocks* in it: *Ars.*, CAMPH., *cupr.*, *ipec.*, *jatroph.*, PHOS., PHOS. AC., *secal.*, VERAT. If there is inflammation, consult also, Acon., bry., and rhus.

Rice-water stools, or *watery*, *greyish*, *whitish* and *flocculent* stools, with great *thirst:* ARS., *camph.*, *cupr.*, ipec., PHOS., PHOS. AC., VERAT. If in the *inflammatory* variety, or in the 4th stage: acon., bry., or rhus.

Stools *whitish:* Acon., ars., *camph.*, bell., *cham.*, *chin.*, cupr., *ipec.*, *jat.*, merc., nux, PHOS., PHOS. AC., sec., sulph., *verat.*

Watery and *white flocky* stools, with *cramps* and *thirst:* Acon., *ars.*, bry., CAMPH., CUPR., ipec., *phos.*, *phos. ac.*, rhus SEC., VERAT.

Watery and *white-flocky* stools, with *clonic spasms*, (spasmodic movements) and *thirst:* Acon., ARS., bry., CAMPH., CUPR., ipec., *phos.*, *phos. ac.*, SEC., VERAT.

Whitish Flocks in *serous* stools, with *pulse* scarcely perceptible: Acon., Ars., bry., Camph., Phos. ac., rhus Sec., Verat.

Liquid stools, with *white* flocks and grains, having the consistence and color of *tallow*: PHOS.

Stools *yellowish*: Ars., *cham*, ipec., *merc.*, Phos., Phos. ac., puls, tart. *verat.*

Yellowish stools, especially in an early stage of the disease: Ars., *cham.*, *ipec.*, *merc.*, Phos., PHOS. AC., tart., Verat.

URINE.

Retention of urine: Camph., Canth., lach., op, plumb., Verat.

Retention of Urine, with ineffectual *desire* to urinate; at the commencement of the stage of *reaction*: CANTH., *verat.*

Urine *scantily* secreted, or *suppressed*: *Ars. camph.*, Carb. v., Cupr., ipec., Sec., stram., VERAT.

The *same symptom* in the consecutive *fever*: Bell., *carb. v.*, Rhus, *stram.*

Secretion of urine *diminished*; with *cramps* in the *calves* of the *legs*: *Ars.*, calc., Camph., cann., *carb. v.*, coff., coloc., con., CUPR., *graph.*, *hyos.*, lach., lyc., merc., natr., *nux*, petr., rhus, *sec.*, sep., sil., sulph., Verat.

VOICE.

Voice *hoarse*: *Ars.*, bell., bry., calc., *camph.*, CARB. V., caus., cham., chin., *cic.*, *cupr.*, dros., graph., hep., *laur.*, merc., natr., *natr. m.*, nux, Phos., *phos. ac.*, puls., rhus, *sec.*, spong., sulph., Verat.

Voice *hoarse*; *face cholerie*: Ars., *camph.*, Carb. v., Cupr., *laur.*, Phos., *phos. ac.*, rhus, *sec.*, Verat.

Voice *lost*, (aphonia): Ant., bell., CARB. V., caus., cham., chin., *cupr.*, dros., hep., kal., lach., *laur.*, merc., *natr. m.*, nux, petr., Phos., puls., sep., sil., spong., stann., sulph., Verat.

CHEST.

Anguish in the chest: Acon., ARS., bell., bry., *camph.*, *carb. v.*, cic., Cupr., hydrocyan., *ipec.*, Jatroph., *laur.*, *natr. m.*, *phos.*, Phos. ac., *rhus*, stram., VERAT.

Breath cold: CARB. V. And, according to some clinical observations, *ars.*, *camph.*, *verat.*

Constriction (spasmodic) *of the chest:* CAMPH., caus., CUPR., fer., IPEC., lach., nitr. ac., *nux*, op., PHOS., phos. ac., puls., spig., *stram.* sulph. VERAT.

Cramps or tonic spasms in the chest: ARS., bell., CAMPH., caus., CIC., CUPR., fer., graph., hyos., IPEC., kal., *merc.*, nux, op., PHOS., *phos. ac.*, puls., SEC., sep., *stram.*, sulph., VERAT.

Cramps in the muscles of the chest, with continual *vomitings*, and with the *eyes turned upwards:* CAMPH., CIC., VERAT.

Respiration laborious; cold and *blue skin:* ARS., CAMPH., CARB. V., CUPR., ipec., *sec.*, VERAT.

SUPERIOR EXTREMITIES.

Cramps in the *upper arms: Phos. ac.* SEC.

Cramps in the *forearms: Laur. phos. ac.*, SEC.

Cramps in the *wrist: Phos. ac.*

Coldness of the *hands:* Acon., bell., *cham.*, *ipec.*, *natr. m.*, nux, petr., *phos.*, sulph., *tart.*, VERAT.

Cramps in the *hands: Bell.* calc., cann., coloc., graph., *laur.*, *phos. ac.*, SEC., stram.

Cramps in the *fingers:* Arn., *ars.*, *calc.*, *cann.*, coff., dros., fer., lyc., nux, *phos.*, *phos. ac.*, SEC., *stann.*, staph., sulph., VERAT.

INFERIOR EXTREMITIES.

Cramps in the *nates:* VERAT.

Cramps in the *hips: Coloc.*, *phos. ac.*

Cramps in the *thighs:* CAMPH., *cann.*, *hyos.*, *ipec.*, merc., petr., *phos ac.*, rhus, sep., VERAT.

Cramps in the *hams: Calc.*, *cann.*, *phos.*

Cramps in the *legs: Carb. v.*, coloc., CUPR., JAT., *phos. ac.*

Cramps in the *calves* of the *legs: Ars.*, bry., calc., CAMPH., cann., *carb. v.*, cham., coff., coloc., CUPR., graph., *hyos.*, JAT., lach., lyc., merc., natr., nitr. ac., *nux*, petr., PHOS., *rhus*, *sec.*, sep., sil., *sol. n.*, staph., *sulph.*, *tart.*, VERAT.

Cramps in the calves of the legs, with burning heat in the stomach, or pit of stomach: ARS., CAMPH., PHOS.

Cramps in the *calves* of the *legs*, with diminished secretion of *urine*: *Ars.*, calc., CAMPH., cann., *carb. v.* caff., coloc., CUPR., *graph.*, *hyos.*, lach., lyc., magn., merc., natr., *nux*, petr., rhus, *sec.*, sep., sil., staph., *sulph.*, VERAT.

Cramps in the *calves*; *coldness* of the *feet*: Calc., graph., lach., lyc., merc., natr., nitr. ac., petr., Phos., *rhus rad.*, sep., sil., *sulph.*, *tart.*, VERAT.

Coldness of the feet: Acon., bell., *calc.*, caus., *dig.*, *graph.*, *ipec.*, *kal.*, lach., lyc., merc., *natr.*, *natr. m.*, *nitr. ac.*, petr., Phos., plat., plumb., *rhod.*, *rhus rad.*, *sep.*, *sil.*, *sulph.*, *tart.*, Verat.

Cramps in the *feet*: CAMPH., caus., graph., lyc., natr., nux., *sec.*, stram., sulph.

Cramps in the feet, with burning in the stomach, or pit of stomach: CAMPH.

Cramps in the *soles* of the feet: Calc., *carb. v.*, coff., fer., hep., petr., *phos. ac.*, plumb., *sec.*, sil., staph., sulph.

Cramps in the *toes*: Calc., fer., hep., lyç., merc., nux, *phos. ac.*, *sec.*, sulph.

SKIN.

Blueness of the skin: Acon., arn., Ars., *bell.*, bry., calc., *camph.*, Carb. v., Cupr., *dig.*, *lach.*, merc., natr. m., nux., *op.*, *phos.*, *phos. ac.*, plumb., puls., rhus, Sec., sil., spong., thuj., VERAT.

Coldness of the skin: Acon., ant., arn., *ars.*, *bell.*, bry., calc., Camph., cann., canth., Carb. v., *caus.*, cham., chin., *cic.*, *cupr.*, dros., dulc., fer., graph., hell., hep., hyos., ign., Ipec., kal., lach., *laur.*, *lyc.*, *merc.*, *mez.*, natr., *natr. m.*, nitr. ac., *nux*, op., petr., Phos., *phos. ac.*, plumb., puls., *rhus*, sabad., sabin., *sec.*, sep., sil., spig., spong., stann., staph., *stram.*, *sulph.*, *tart.*, thuj., VERAT.

The medicines which correspond both to *coldness* and *blueness* (of the skin), respectively or collectively, are: Acon., arn., Ars., *bell.*, bry., calc., Camph., Carb. v., Cupr., *lach.*, merc., natr. m., nux, op., Phos., Phos. ac., plumb., puls., rhus, Sec., sil., spong., thuj., VERAT.

Skin *cold* and *bluish*, and covered with *cold perspiration*: ARS., camph., *carb. v.*, CUPR., ipec., *secal.*, VERAT.

Coldness of the skin, with mental indifference or tranquillity: ARS, ipec., NATR. M., VERAT.

Withered or *wrinkled* skin: *Ant.*, ARS., bry., calc., *camph.*, cham., *chin.*, CUPR., fer., graph., hell., hyos., iod., kal., *lyc.*, merc., mur. ac., nux, *phos.*, PHOS. AC., rheum., SEC., *sep.*, *sil.*, spig., spong., stram., sulph., VERAT.

The medicines which correspond, respectively or collectively, to *blueness*, *coldness* and *shrivelled* state of the skin, are: ARS., bry., calc., CAMPH., CUPR., merc., nux, PHOS., PHOS. AC., SEC., sil., spong., VERAT.

The medicines which, on the ground of clinical experience, have been more especially recommended for this combination of symptoms, in the stage of collapse in cholera, are: ARS., CAMPH., CARB. V., CUPR., *hydrocy.*, jat., SEC., VERAT.

PERSPIRATION AND PULSE.

Cold perspiration: Acon., ARS., bell., bry., calc., CAMPH., canth., CARB. V., cham., chin., cin., coff., CUPR., dulc., hell., hep., hyos., ign., IPEC., lach., lyc., merc., natr., nitr. ac., nux, op., petr., *phos.*, *phos. ac.*, plumb., puls., rheum, rhus, sabad., SEC., sep., sil., spig., stram., sulph., thuj., *tart.*, VERAT.

Viscid, clammy, perspiration: ARS. *camph.* daph., fer., hep., *jat.*, lach., lyc., merc., nux, *phos.*, *phos. ac.*, plumb., *sec.*, VERAT.

Pulse feeble and *frequent:* *Ars.*, CARB. V., *lach.*, nux, rhus rad.

Pulse Feeble and *Slow*, in the 1*st stage*: CAMPH., cann., dig., LAUR., *merc.*, puls., *rhus. rad.*, VERAT.

Pulse Feeble and *Slow*, in the 4th *stage:* *Camph.*, cann., dig., *laur.*, *merc.*, *puls.*, R. RAD., VERAT.

Pulse *feeble* and *small:* ARS., CAMPH., chin., dig., LACH., *nux*, PHOS. AC., puls., RHUS, VERAT.

Pulse scarcely perceptible, with *watery* and *white-flocky stools:* Acon., ARS., bry., CAMPH., PHOS. AC., rhus, SEC., VERAT.

GENERAL AND MISCELLANEOUS SYMPTOMS.

Internal *burning*, and *tossing*, with *fear of death:* ARS.

Burnings in the *stomach* and *abdomen*, with *anguish* and *tossing:* ARS., CAMPH.

Cholera followed by *cerebral* and abdominal affections: BELL.

Cramps or other *Spasms* at *night: Ars*, *camph.*, calc., cin., CUPR., hyos., *ipec.*, kal., lyc., merc., op., SEC.

Cramps in the *stomach* and *extremities*, with *coldness of the body* in an early stage, with but little diarrhœa: CAMPH

Clonic Spasms, (convulsions): *Ars.*, *Bell.*, bry., calc., CAMPH., canth., *carb. v.*, caus., cham., *cic.*, con., CUPR., *hyos.*, ign., *ipec*, cal., lyc., merc., *natr. m.*, op., *phos.*, phos. ac., plat., rhus., SEC., sep., sil., stann., STRAM., tart., sulph., VERAT.

Severe clonic Spasms, with but little diarrhœa or vomiting: *Ars.*, CAMPH., CUPR., ipec., *sec.*, VERAT.

Tonic Spasms, (Tetanus, Cramps, &c.): *Ars.*, *bell.*, caus., *cham.*, CIC., CUPR., ign., *ipec.*, lyc., merc., *petr.*, *phos.*, *plat.*, rhus, SEC., sep., *stram.*, sulph., VERAT.

Severe *tonic Spasms*, with but little diarrhœa or vomiting: CAMPH., CUPR., ipec., SEC., VERAT.

Cramps or other *Spasms*, in the *extremities* or elsewhere, with weight, pressive *pain* or *aching*, at the *pit* of the *stomach:* CAMPH., CUPR., natr. m., *phos.*, *phos. ac.*, *sec.*, *tart.*, VERAT.

Spasms of the extremities, with *painful sensibility* of the *pit* of the *stomach: Ars.* CAMPH., CUPR., natr. m., *phos.*, *phos. ac.*, tart., VERAT.

Collapse, without previous or present vomiting or diarrhœa: CAMPH., CARB. v., *hydrocy.*, laur., VERAT.

Collapse almost or quite *complete*, and without diarrhœa, vomiting or spasms: Camph., CARB. V., HYDROCY., *laur.*, verat.

Excessive and sudden *debility: Ars.*, carb. v., CUPR., *ipec.*, lach., *laur.*, nux, PHOS., PHOS. AC., *sec*, VERAT.

The patient *worse after midnight*, or early in the *morning:* Acon., ARS., bell., canth., CARB. v., CUPR., kal.. *lach.*, merc., natr., *natr. m.*, *nux*, *petr.*, PHOS., PHOS. AC., RHUS., *sec.*, stram., sulph., *tart.*, VERAT.

The patient made *worse by movement:* Acon., Ars., Bell., *bry.*, Camph., canth., carb v., cic., Cupr., dig., hyos., Ipec , kal., lach., *laur.*, *merc.*, *natr. m.*, *nux*, *petr.*, Phos., Phos. ac., plumb., *rhus*, *rad.*, Sec., stram., sulph., *tart.*, Verat.

ADDENDA.

Vertigo with *nausea* and *thirst:* VERAT.

Coldness of the Nose: Arn., bell., plumb., *Verat.*

Coldness of the Nose and Hands: Bell., VERAT.

Anxiety, distension and pressure at the pit of the stomach: *Ars.*

Sensibility and *Swelling* of the pit of the Stomach: Hep., lyc . *natr. m.*, *sulph.*

Throbbings in the Abdomen: Caps. ign. op. plumb. sang. *tart.*

CHAPTER X.

GASTRIC AND INTESTINAL REPERTORY.

AUXILIARY TO THE CHOLERA REPERTORY, AND ADAPTED TO VOMITING AND DIARRHŒA IN GENERAL, AND TO CHOLERA INFANTUM AND DYSENTERY.

EXPLANATION OF THE USE OF THE REPERTORY.

The arrangement of the symptoms of each section, is in general alphabetical.

The mode of obtaining the remedy for a group, is the same in this, as in the Cholera Repertory. The medicines seldom required, are here omitted. The emphasis in Chapter X., has no special reference to the Cholera; but in the treatment of this disease, this chapter may be consulted, when any case presents symptoms contained in this, but not in the Cholera Repertory; and that Repertory may be used as auxiliary to this and in general practice; for the medicines there enumerated apply to the symptoms, in whatever disease they may occur.

The 30th, will in general be a suitable dilution for most medicines, in ordinary gastric and intestinal diseases, for which this Repertory (Chap. X.) is more especially constructed.

VOMITING IN GENERAL.

Acon., ant., arn., *ars.*, bell., *bry.*, calc., camph., cann., canth., carb. v., *cham.*, chin , cic., cin.. coff., colch., coloc., *cupr.*, dros., dulc , *fer.*, graph., hep., hyos., ign., *ipec.*, lach., laur., lyc., merc., natr. m., nitr. ac , *nux*, phos., plumb., *puls.*, sec., sep , *sil.*, stann., stram , *sulph.*, tart., *verat.*

CHARACTER OF THE VOMITING.

Vomiting; Acrid: Arg., ipec.

—— Bilious, bitter: *Acon.*, *ant.*, *ars.*, *bry.*, camph., *cann.*, *colch.*, *cupr* , *dros.*, *grat* , *ipec* , lach., *merc.*, *nux*, *phos.*, *puls.*, *sec.*, *sep.*, stann., stram , sulph., *verat.*

Vomiting, Bitterish-Sour: Grat., ipec., puls.
—— Blackish: *Ars.*, calc., chin., hell., lau., *nux*, phos., plumb., sec., sulph., *verat.*
—— of Blood: *Acon.*, arn., ars., bell., *bry.*, calc., camph., canth., *carb. v.*, caus., chin., cupr., dros., *fer.*, hep., *hyos.*, *lach.*, lyc., *mez.*, *nux*, op., *phos.*, plumb., puls., sulph., *verat.*, zinc.
—— of Blood Clotted: Arn., caus.
Vomiting of Blood; sour regurgitations: Ars., calc., *carb. v.*, *lyc.*, *nux*, phos., plumb., puls., *sulph.*
Vomiting Brownish: Ars., bis.
Vomiting of what has been Drank: Acon., ant., arn., *ars.*, *bry.*, cham., chin., dulc., *ipec.*, nux, puls., sec., sil., sulph., tart., verat.
—— of what has been Eaten: Ant., *ars.*, bell., *bry.*, calc., chin., colch., coloc., cupr., dros., *fer.*, hyos., ign., *ipec.*, lach., laur., lyc., *natr. m.*, *nux*, phos., plumb., *puls.*, sep., sil., stann., *sulph.*, *verat.*
—— of Excrement: Bell., bry., nux., *op.*, plumb.
—— Frothy: Æth., *verat.*
—— Gelatinous: *Ipec.*
—— Green: Acon., *ars.*, *cann.*, *ipec.*, lach., phos., *plumb.*, puls.. *verat.*
—— Milky. Æth.
—— of Milk used: *Æth.*, samb.
—— of Mucus: *Acon.*, æth., *ars.*, *bell.*, *bor.*, bry., *cham.*, *chin.*, cupr, *dig.*, dros., *dulc.*, hyos., *ipec.*, lach., *merc.*, *nux*, phos., *puls.*, *sulph.*, *verat.*
—— of Bloody Mucus: Acon., hep., hyos., lach., nitr.
—— of Green Mucus: *Acon.*, *ars.*, *ipec.*, lach., phos., *puls.*, *verat.*
—— Painful: *Asar.*, tart.
—— Periodical: Cupr., nux.
—— Salt: Magn., natr. s.
Vomiting Sour: Ars.. bell., bor., *calc.*, *caus.*, cham., chin., fer., graph, hep., ipec., lyc., *nux.*, *phos.*, phos. ac., *puls.*, sass., stram., *sulph.*, tab, tart., thuj., verat.
—— Violent: *Ars.*, bell., cupr., *iod.*, *lach.*, nux, *plumb.*, *tart.*, *verat.*
—— Watery: Ars., bell., *caus.*, chin., cupr., hyos., *jat.*, magn., sil., stann., stram., sulph. ac., tab., *verat.*
—— Yellowish: Ars., iod., oleand., plumb.
—— Yellow, with tinge of Green: Oleand., verat.

CAUSES OR CONDITIONS OF THE VOMITING.

Vomiting after Acids: Fer.
—— after Bread: Nitr. ac.
—— from the motion of a Carriage: *Ars.*, *cocc.*, nux, petr., sil, sulph.
—— after a Chill: Bell.

Vomiting, after Drinking: *Arn.*, *ars.*, bry., *nux*, *puls.*, sil.
—— relieved by Drinking: *Cupr.*
—— bitter after Drinking: *Ars*, *nux*, sil, *verat.*
Vomiting after Eating: *Ars.*, *calc.*, *fer.*, iod., ipec., lach., *nux*, phos., *puls.*, *sep.*, *sil.*, stann., sulph., *verat.*
—— Evening (in the): Bell., bry., phos., puls., sulph.
—— Morning (in the): Bar. m., dig., dros., *nux.*, sil., sulph.
—— Night (at): Ars., bry., caus., dig., dros., *fer.*, lyc., merc., mur. ac., nux, phos, *puls.*, sulph., verat.
—— in Pregnancy: Acon., ars., *con.*, fer., *ipec.*, kreos., lach., magn. m., natr. m., n. mos., nux, petr., phos., *puls.*, sep., verat.
Vomiting after Smoking or Stooping: Ipec.
—— from the motion of a Ship: *Ars*, *cocc.*, nux, petr., sil., sulph.
—— after Sucking: Sil.

CONCOMITANTS OF THE VOMITING.

Vomiting with:
—— Anxiety: Ant., ars., nux.
—— offensive Breath: *Ipec.*
—— Choking: Hyos.
—— Colic: Ars., bry., nux, plumb., *puls.*, stram., tart., verat.
—— Convulsions: Ant., *cupr.*, hyos., merc.
—— Cries: Ars.
—— fear of Death: Ars.
—— Diarrhœa: Æth., ant., *ars.*, bell., coloc., *cupr.*, *jat.*, *ipec.*, lach., phos., rheum., stram., tart., *verat.*
—— pains in the Ears: Puls.
—— Eructations: Caus., mur. ac.
—— Eyes convulsed: Cic.
—— Face, pale: *Puls.*, tart.
—— perspiration on the Face: Camph., sulph.
—— Feet, cold: Kreos, phos.
—— Feet, numb: Phos.
—— Hands, cold: Kreos., phos., verat.
—— Hands, hot: Verat.
—— Hands, numb: Phos.
—— Heat: *Ars.*, bell., ipec., verat.
—— Hiccough: Bry.
—— Legs, cramped: Nux.
—— desire to lie down: *Verat.*
—— Nausea: Nux, sulph., *verat.*
—— Pain in the back: Puls.
—— Pain in the stomach: Ars., *cupr.*, hyos., ipec., lach., *op.*, *phos.*, plumb., sulph., tart., verat.
—— Perspiration: *Ipec.*, sulph.

Vomiting, with Perspiration, cold: Camph.
—— Rumbling: Puls.
—— Shivering: Bry., *phos.*, *puls.*, tart., sulph.
—— Shivering in the evening: Bry., *phos.*, sulph.
—— Shuddering: Verat.
—— Sight, obscure: Lach.
—— Sleepiness: *Tart.*
—— Taste, bitter: *Puls.*
—— Thirst: *Ipec.*
—— Throat, burning: Arg., puls.
—— Trembling: Nux, tart.
—— Vertigo: Hyos., natr. s.
—— Weakness: *Ars.*, hyos., *ipec.*, phos., *verat.*

SENSATIONS (PAINS, &c.,) AT THE STOMACH AND PIT OF THE STOMACH.

Burning in the pit of the stomach: Acon., ant., ars., bell., bry., laur., merc., nux, phos., sec., sep., sil. sulph., verat.

—— In the stomach: *Ars.*, bell., *bry.*, camph., *canth.*, *caps.*, *carb. v.*, cham., cic., graph., ign., *laur.*, *merc.*, merc. c., *nitr.*, *nux*, *phos.*, phos. ac., *sabad.*, *sec.*, *sep.*, *sulph.*, verat.

Cold sensation in the Stomach or pit: *Ars.*, bell., ign., lach., laur., phos., phos. ac., rhus, sulph.

Cramp: [See spasmodic pains.]

Sensation of *Emptiness* in the Stomach: Ant., ign., petr., sep., tart., verat.

Sensation of *Fulness* in the Stomach and pit: *Arn.*, *bar. c.*, bell., carb. v., cham., *grat.*, *hell.*, *kal.*, *lyc.*, nux, petr., *phos.*, *sulph.*

—— after a meal: Also, *chin.*, *merc.*, *puls.*, *sep.*, *sil.*

Pressure in the pit of the stomach: Acon., *arn.*, *ars.*, *bell.*, camph., *cham.*, chin., coff., coloc., cupr., hep., ign., merc., *natr. m.*, *nitr.*, *nux*, *phos.*, *phos. ac.*, *prun.*, *puls.*, *ran.*, *ran. sc.*, *rhod.*, *rhus*, *sep.*, *stann.*, *sulph.*, *tart.*, *verat.*

—— in the stomach: *Acon.*, *agar.*, *anac.*, *arn.*, *ars.*, *bar. c.*, *bell.*, *bis.*, *bry.*, *calc.*, canth., *carb. an.*, *carb. v.*, *cham.*, *chin.*, *cic.*, coff., coloc., *fer.*, *graph.*, *grat.*, *hep.*, *iod.*, ipec., *lach.*, *laur.*, *led.*, *lyc.*, *merc.*, *mez.*, *mosch.*, *natr.*, *natr. m.*, *nux*, *par.*, *petr.*, *phos.*, *plat.*, *plumb.*, puls., *rhod.*, rhus, *sabin.*, *sec.*, *san.*, *sep.*, *sil.*, spig., *squill.*, *stann.*, stram., *sulph.*, *tart.*

Shootings in the Pit of the Stomach: *Arn.*, bell., *bry.*, *kal.*, *nit. ac.*, phos., puls., rhus, sep., sulph., tart.

—— In the stomach: Bell., *bry.*, coff., ign., *kal.*, plat., sep., sulph.

Spasmodic pains in the stomach: *Ant.*, ars., bell., *bis.*, *bry.*, *calc.*, *carb. a.*, *carb. v.*, *caus.*, *cham.*, *chin.*, *cocc.*, *coff.*, *con.*, cupr., *fer.*, *graph.*, *hyos.*, *kal.*, *lach.*, *lyc.*, merc., *natr. m.*, *nux*, phos., *puls.*, sec., *sep.*, *sulph.*, verat.

Swelling of the pit of the stomach: Acon., calc., hep., lyc., sulph.

Sensation of Swelling there: Bry..

Tenderness of the stomach and region of the stomach: Am. c., am. m., ant., ars., bar. c., bry., calc., camph., canth., carb. v., caus., colch., coloc., hep., hyos., kreos., *lach.*, lyc., magn. m., merc., natr., natr. m., nux, ol. an., phos., phos. ac., puls., *rhus rad.*, sil., spong., stann., sulph., sulph. ac., tart., tereb., verat.

Tension in the Pit of the stomach: Acon., ant., cham., *nux.*

—— in the Stomach: Acon., bry., carb. v., kal., merc., staph.

Throbbings in the region of the stomach: Acon., bell., kal., *puls.*, rhus, sep., sulph., tart., thuy.

DIARRHŒA IN GENERAL.

Acon., alum., am. m., ant., arn., *ars.*, bell., bor., bry., *calc.*, carb. v., *cham.*, *chin.*, cic., coff., coloc., con., cupr., dig., dros., dulc., fer., graph., hep., hyos., ign., ipec., *lach.*, laur., lyc., *merc.*, natr. m., nitr. ac., nux, petr., *phos.*, *phos. ac.*, *puls.*, rheum., *rhus*, sep., sil., stram., *sulph.*, sulph. ac., *verat.*

COLOR OF THE FÆCES.

Color, Black: *Ars.*, bry., calc., camph., *chin.*, ipec., merc., nux, op., phos., stram., sulph., sulph. ac., verat.

—— Brownish: Ars., camph., dulc., magn., magn. m., merc. c., rheum., rhus rad., sulph., verat.

—— Clay-like: Calc., hep.

—— Greyish: Merc., phos., phos. ac., rheum.

—— Greenish: *Ars.*, *bell.*, *cham.*, coloc., dulc., hep., ipec., magn., magn. m., *merc.*, merc. c., nux, *phos.*, phos. ac., *puls.*, rheum., sep., *sulph.*, sulph. ac., *verat.*

—— Pale: Carb. v., lyc.

—— Whitish: *Acon.*, ars., calc., caus., *cham.*, *chin.*, *colch.*, *cop.*, *dig.*, *hep.*, *ign.*, iod., nux, phos., phos. ac., *puls.*, rhus, spig., spong., *sulph.*

—— White, like milk: Arn., *bell.*, dulc., merc., nux, rheum.

—— White like flocks: Vide, *Cholera Repertory.*

—— White, in streaks: Rhus tox.

—— Yellowish: *Ars.*, calc., *cham.*, chin., cocc., coloc., ign., ipec., merc., phos., plumb., puls., sulph., terb.

—— Yellow in streaks: Rhus tox.

ODOR OF THE FÆCES.

Odor:

—— Corpse-like: Sil., carb. v.

—— Fœtid: Ars., calc., cham., coloc., lach., merc., merc.

c., nitr. ac., nux., op., phos. ac., plumb., rheum., sep., squill., sulph., sulph. ac., tab.

Odor, Putrid: Ars., bry., carb. v., cham., chin., coloc., graph., *merc.*, nitr. ac., nux., sep., sulph., sulph ac.

—— Sour: Arn., calc., coloc., graph., magn., *merc.*, rheum., sep., sulph.

COMPOSITION AND CONSISTENCE OF THE FÆCES.

Fæces; acrid: Ars., cham., fer., lach., *merc.*, puls., sass., verat.

—— Bilious: Ars., dulc., ipec., *merc.*, merc. c., puls.

—— Bloody: Arn., ars., caps., carb. v., colch., coloc., dulc., *ipec.*, lach., *merc.*, merc. c., *nitr. ac*, *nux.*

—— coated with Blood: Con., magn. m., nux, squill., thuy.

—— Burning: Ars., lach., *merc.*

—— Clay-like: Calc.

—— Corrosive: See *Acrid.*

—— not Digested: Arn., ars., bry., calc., cham., chin., con., fer., lach., merc., nitr. ac., oleand., phos., phos. ac., squill., sulph.

—— not Digested at night, or after meals: *Chin.*

—— Fermented: Ipec., sabad.

—— Frothy: Calc., coloc., iod., lach., merc., op., rhus., sulph. ac.

—— Gelatinous: Rhus, sep.

—— Purulent: *Arn.* bell., *calc.*, *canth*, *chin.*, clem., cocc., con., ignat., iod., kal., *lyc.*, *merc.*, nux, petr., *puls.*, sabin., *sep.*, *sil.*, *sulph.*

—— Slimy: *Ang.*, arn., *ars.*, *bell.*, caps., *carb. v.*, *cham.*, *chin.*, coloc., *dulc.*, *fer.*, *graph*, hell., iod., ipec., kal., *merc.*, nitr. ac., *nux phos.*, phos. ac., *puls.*, *rheum.*, *rhus.*, *sec.*, *sep.*, *squill.*, *stann.*, *sulph.*, *tart.*, verat.

—— Viscous; sticky: Calc., carb. v., caus. hep., lach., *merc.*, nux, plumb., sass., verat.

—— Watery: Acon., ant., arn., *ars.*, bell., *calc.*, *cham.*, *chin.*, *fer.*, *hyos.*, jat., ipec., *lach.*, *nux*, petr., phos., phos. ac., *puls.*, *rhus.*, *sec.*, sulph., tart., verat.

CAUSES, OR CONDITIONS OF DIARRHŒA.

Diarrhœa:

—— from Acid things: Lach.

—— after taking Cold: *Bell*, *bry.*, caus., *cham.*, chin., *dulc.* *merc.*, *n-mos.*, nux, puls., sulph., verat.

—— in the Coolness of the evening: *Merc.*

—— in Damp weather: Lach., rhod.

—— Day and night: Sulph.

—— after Drinking: *Ars.*, cin.

Diarrhœa, in the Evening: Caus., kal., lach., merc.
—— in Feeble persons: Chin., fer., rhus, phos. ac., sec.
—— after Fruits: Chin., lach., rhod.
—— from Grief: Ign.
—— from Indigestion: Ant., coff., ipec., puls., nux.
—— after a Meal: Ars., chin., lach., verat.
—— after Milk: Bry., lyc., sep., sulph.
—— in the Morning: Bry.
—— at Night: *Ars*, bry., *cham.*, *chin.*, dulc., lach., *merc.*, *mosch.*, *puls.*, *rhus*, *sulph.*, verat.
—— of Old persons: Ant., bry., phos., sec.
—— of Pregnant females: Ant., dulc., hyos., lyc., petr., phos., sep., sulph.
—— of Scrofulous persons: Ars., bar. c., *calc.*, chin., *dulc.*, *lyc.*, *sep.*, *sil.*, *sulph.*
—— when sleeping: Arn., puls., rhus.
—— during warm weather: Lach.

CONCOMITANTS OF DIARRHŒA.

Diarrhœa with:
—— Abdomen distended: Graph., sulph., verat.
—— Anguish: Ant., lach., merc.
—— excoriation of the Anus: Cham., merc., sass.
—— Colic, cutting: Acon., *agar.*, *ang.*, *ant.*, *ars.*, *asa.*, *bar. c.*, *bry.*, *cann.*, *canth.*, *cham.*, *coloc.*, dulc., hep., *ipec.*, lach., *merc.*, *merc. c.*, *mez.*, *nux*, *petr.*, *puls.*, *rat.*, *rheum*, *rhus*, *stront.*, *sulph.*, *verat.*
—— alternately with Constipation: Bry., lach., nux, rhus.
—— with Cries and tears, in children: Carb. v., *cham.*, *ipec.*, rheum, sulph.
—— *Debility*: *Ars.*, *chin.*, *ipec.*, phos., sep., *verat.*
—— Eructations: Con., dulc., merc.
—— Heat: Merc.
—— pain in the Limbs: Am. m., rhus.
—— pain in the Loins: Nux.
—— Nausea: Ars., bell., ip., lach., *merc.*
—— cold Perspiration on the face: Merc.
—— Shiverings: *merc.*, *puls.*, *sulph.*
—— pain in the Stomach: Bell., bry.
—— Tenesmus: Ars., ipec., lach., *merc.*, nux, rheum, rhus, sulph.
—— Thirst: Ars., dulc.
—— Vomitings: *Ars.*, bell., coloc., cupr., dulc., *ipec.*, lach., phos., rheum, stram., tart., *verat.*

GROUPS OF DIARRHŒIC SYMPTOMS.

Stool, part Black; part Green: *Ars.*, ipec., *merc.*, phos., sulph. ac., *verat.*

CPSIA information can be obtained at www.ICGtesting.com
Printed in the USA
237724LV00004B/78/P

9 781145 503